# 62Q

## Sixty-two Questions For Your Dominant

## MICHAEL MAKAI

Copyright © 2014 Michael Makai

All rights reserved.

ISBN-13: 978-1502775948
ISBN-10: 1502775948

# DEDICATION

This book is for the submissives.

May you find lasting happiness

with your One.

# Table of Contents

Table of Contents ..................................................................................... 5
Introduction .............................................................................................. 7
    A Prefatory Note on Gender Bias ..................................................... 10
Chapter 1: Interviewing ......................................................................... 11
    Stupid Questions - There Are Some ................................................. 13
    Ask Open-ended Questions ............................................................... 14
    Ask for *Unnecessary* Explanations .................................................. 15
    Dare to Ask For Specifics .................................................................. 17
    Get a Second Opinion ....................................................................... 17
    Don't Stop Wondering ...................................................................... 18
Chapter 2: Before You Meet .................................................................. 20
    New Relationship Energy (NRE) ..................................................... 21
Chapter 3: Before a Collar ................................................................... 154
Chapter 4: After the Collar .................................................................. 166
Chapter 5: Epilogue .............................................................................. 180
Appendix A: Bonus Questions ............................................................. 184
Appendix B: Glossary ........................................................................... 190
Appendix C: About the Author ............................................................ 197

Michael Makai

# Introduction

"Why didn't I listen to my friends when they told me to be careful? Why didn't I trust my instincts when they told me that something about him wasn't right? Why did I believe all of the bullshit explanations he fed me all these months? How could I have been so incredibly stupid? That's it! I'm leaving the BDSM lifestyle forever!"

Sound familiar? Of *course* it does.

If it doesn't sound like a familiar refrain from your own life, you probably know more than one person who has wailed some variation of the above, and probably on more than one occasion. It's a sad fact of life and relationships that most of us fail to take even the most rudimentary steps needed to help us navigate through the certain minefields of BDSM dating and relationships.

We're going to fix that, at least as it applies to your little corner of the universe. I'm going to teach you to interview like a pro, and you'll learn to do it in such a way that your prospective Dominant probably won't even realize that he or she is, in reality, interviewing for a job.

I'm not *only* going to give you the best and most useful questions that every submissive should be asking a prospective Dominant, but I am also going to give you the necessary follow-up questions and tell you why you need to ask them. I'm also going to explain how you should interpret your prospective Dominant's responses and what you should do about it.

What makes me an authority on the art of interviewing prospective Dominants, particularly considering the fact that I happen to be a Dominant, myself?

Good question.

I have over twenty years of experience interviewing and counseling troops while on military active duty. I was trained by the best of the best in the art of interrogation. I've also been a small-business owner and corporate executive who did quite a bit of hiring, firing, and interviewing.

As a Dominant, I've been interviewing, mentoring, and training both Doms and subs for over thirty-seven years.

One thing I've learned in that time is that you won't get the answers you need if you don't ask the right questions.

I've also learned that it is simply a part of human nature to reveal only the things about ourselves that are flattering or useful. Recent studies have shown that close to 88% of all online social media profiles contain significant amounts of outright deception.

I've learned that many people will attempt to compensate for their lack of knowledge or experience by bluffing. You must learn to *call* their bluff and do it in a way that doesn't put you at risk of being outed, ostracized, injured or killed.

If you are reading this book, chances are you were drawn to it because you've already learned some painful lessons about the pitfalls of finding a partner in the BDSM lifestyle.

People lie. Face it: There are a *lot* of people out there who will exploit and use you for their own sexual gratification, financial opportunism, or simple sadistic pleasure. Some of these cretins are extremely good at what they do. Many have been doing it successfully for years.

Why do they do it? They do it because they *can* and because it *works*.

If you were a victim of one of these deceptive twat-waffles, you probably weren't his first victim and you are definitely not going to be his last. There will always be a steady stream of fresh, naive, and inexperienced new submissives in the throes of sub-frenzy who are eager to be collared, despite not having the foggiest notion of who it really is holding the leash.

We can't fix that. Sure, you can try to expose some of them, but for every exploitative creep you expose there will be a thousand more waiting in the shadows for their chance. Realistically, it's practically impossible to warn others about some of these jerks. After all, you were probably warned. Did you listen?

I'm guessing, no. You did not. All you can do is educate and protect yourself.

And I'm going to teach you *how*.

## A Prefatory Note on Gender Bias

Throughout this book, I often refer to Dominants with the male pronoun "he" and submissives with the female pronoun *"she."* I follow this practice not because I am a gender bigot or because I believe that all Dominants are (or should be) males or that all submissives are (or should be) females.

I do it because I am a writer who just wants to get my ideas across to my readers without having to resort to the clunky and annoying practice of using "he or she" in every third sentence or using the grammatically incorrect "they or their" in reference to a singular person.

I do it because I prefer that the beauty and efficacy of the English language not be sullied by political correctness or swayed by an agenda for social justice, even when I happen to back that agenda. I fully support the movements for gender equality and transgender rights.

I also *do* believe in the notion that changing the verbiage that we use can be an effective tool in changing people's perceptions and ideas over time. I do *not*, however, believe that this BDSM book is the appropriate place to fight that particular battle.

# Chapter 1: Interviewing

The greatest challenge you will face while interviewing a prospective Dominant is almost always going to be doing it with tact. A Dominant, almost by definition, typically does not enjoy being interrogated, doubted, or challenged in any way. If he senses that you are questioning his *Dom-cred* or personal integrity, there will likely be fireworks, especially if he just happens to be the real deal.

This is probably a good time to mention that interviewing a prospective Dominant shouldn't be reserved solely for the ones that you suspect may be phonies. An interview should be conducted with every Dominant you are considering, regardless of how authentic, charismatic, or experienced he may seem at first blush. An experienced, knowledgeable Dominant will have nothing to fear and no problem cooperating with a tactfully conducted interview. If he does, that should be your very first yellow flag to consider.

As long as we're on the subject of flags, let's now briefly discuss what we mean when we refer to green, yellow, and red flags.

A green flag is a "credibility point." A green flag is something that somehow confirms what your prospective Dominant has told you. It might be his driver's license, a family photograph, or that college diploma hanging on his office wall. It could be as simple as knowing who his friends are or as complicated as calculating the feasibility of his life events timeline. Green flags are always a good thing. The more of them you accumulate the better.

A yellow flag typically references a bit of suspicious information. Often, it will be the result of behavior that simply doesn't seem to make sense or won't add up in any rational way. Other times, it may be a matter of trusting your own personal intuition or *"spidey-*

*senses"* in any given situation. Careful observation and accurate recall of a person's behavior can reveal all sorts of valuable tell-tale clues. Remember, however, that most yellow flags will turn out to be much ado about nothing, in the end.

A red flag is a sure sign of deception or an indicator of a train wreck ahead. Some examples might include learning that your prospective Dominant has been dishonest with you about his experience level, knowledge, gender, location, marital status, or any other significant portions of his life story. Please keep in mind, however, that in the early stages of any relationship, no one owes anyone the kind of sensitive information that can be used to wreak havoc in their personal or professional lives.

He might be comfortable telling you that he works as a carpenter in Cincinnati without giving you the name of the company he works for. That's perfectly reasonable and prudent. On the other hand, if that same guy tells you he's a billionaire in Buenos Aires, that just might be a red flag.

The most important thing to remember here is that he is not obligated to give you the unfiltered, absolute truth about every single thing you ask him. Even if he did, that wouldn't exactly certify him as an honest man; it would more accurately mark him as a complete *moron*. Is that really what you're looking for?

Be careful about assigning a red flag to every falsehood without any real regard for its significance. Not every untruth is unscrupulous, nor is every truth virtuous.

So, how can you interview your prospective Dominant with finesse? How do you exercise such delicacy and tact that he not only tolerates the interview, but enjoys it?

Two words: *genuine interest.* If you really are genuinely interested in him, he will sense it and will likely be thrilled to cooperate. Conversely, if he feels he is being tested or challenged, he will not.

## Stupid Questions - There Are Some

Showing an interest in what your prospective Dominant has to say is just half the battle. If you're too focused on the wrong things, you'll not only get nothing but useless information from the interview, but you'll also end up looking clueless or misinformed. I can honestly say that I've been interviewed hundreds of times over the last thirty-seven years and in at least ninety percent of the time, the submissive conducting the interview ended up botching it.

You're probably wondering, how does something like that happen? *Easy.* You ask incredibly dopey questions that reveal your own ignorance, biases, and naiveté.

The following list contains some actual questions I've been asked by submissives who thought that I was the only one being evaluated during their interview:

Q: What's your favorite safeword?
Me: *"More."*

Q: If I told you I'd do anything to serve you, what would you have me do?
Me: Mow and edge my lawn. You got a weedeater?

Q: Do you think emotions have any place in a D/s relationship?
Me: I suppose it depends on whether or not that's a real Uzi you're packing.

Q: Would you tell me to do things that I don't want to do?

Me: What would be the point of telling you to do things that you are already going to do?

Q: What's your favorite thing to do to a submissive?
Me: I enjoy keeping my sarcasm in check while pretending that she's asking me sensible questions.

Q: What do you do to earn a submissive's respect?
Me: I challenge her to an all-night chicken dance marathon.

Q: Would you mind if I refused to call you *Sir?* I'd prefer to come up with my own little pet name for you.
Me: No problem. As long as you don't mind me calling you "that girl I used to know."

Needless to say, interviewers like that rarely made it past the first round of talks. My point in sharing these awful examples with you is not to frighten you into a state of paralysis, where you're afraid to ask your prospective Dom anything at all. No, my purpose is to emphasize again the importance of asking the right questions. The questions that you ask will tell him far more about *you* than you'll ever learn about *him*.

As you progress through the topics provided in this book, you'll no doubt think of additional questions of your own that you'll want to pose to your prospective Dominant. When you do, try to follow the following rules of thumb.

## Ask Open-ended Questions

An open-ended question is one that cannot be answered with a simple yes or no. The reasoning behind this rule of thumb is simple. A poser will always have a difficult time providing a knowledgeable, coherent answer to an open-ended question, but he will *always* have at least a fifty-fifty chance of correctly answering a yes or no question. Since it usually isn't difficult to figure out which of the two answers is the best guess, a phony can do remarkably well, even when he knows absolutely nothing about the question.

Consider the following two examples, using sample questions about Risk Aware Consensual Kink (RACK), to illustrate this point.

**Close-ended Questioning**

Submissive: Do you follow the RACK principles?
Dominant: Sure!

In this example, it's fairly obvious to the phony Dom that the sub *wants* him to be a believer in RACK.

**Open-ended Questioning**

Submissive: Would you please tell me what you think about RACK?
Dominant: Do you mean those things they tie you to and stretch you with?

In *this* example, it becomes painfully obvious that the Dom doesn't have a clue what RACK is. It's easy to see which type of question reveals more about the prospective Dom's true level of knowledge, experience, and integrity.

People lie. Don't make it *easy* for them.

## Ask for *Unnecessary* Explanations

Be sly. Request explanations for things you already understand. I realize that this may sound just a little counter-intuitive, but it really is the only practical way to successfully gauge the prospective Dom's understanding of certain concepts or processes.

If you ask for explanations for things that you don't understand, how will you ever know if you're getting a real and useful answer, or a completely *bogus* one?

The point of conducting an interview is not to educate yourself on various aspects of the lifestyle. The point of the interview is to make a realistic, useful assessment of your prospective Dominant's knowledge and integrity.

Only after you have deemed him to be sufficiently experienced and qualified to teach you what you wish to know should you try to learn from him. Otherwise, it will simply become a laughably pathetic case of the blind leading the blind.

Here are two examples which demonstrate the difference between necessary and unnecessary explanations.

**Necessary Explanation**
[The submissive does *not* understand TPE.]

Submissive: Would you please explain Total Power Exchange for me?
Dominant: Sure. It means you give all your power to *me*, in exchange for your collar.
Submissive: Ahh! Okay, I thought it might have been a lot more complicated than that.
Dominant: (Preening) Nah. It's simple, really!
(The collective I.Q. in the room drops fifty points.)

**Unnecessary Explanation**
[The submissive understands TPE.]

Submissive: Would you please explain TPE to me?
Dominant: Well, my understanding of it is there is empowerment that passes in each direction in any healthy D/s relationship dynamic. Sometimes it's symmetrical, sometimes, it's asymmetrical.

Submissive: Wow! That sounds rather complicated!
Dominant: Frankly, I'm not sure I understand it very well.
(This couple is off to a great start. Admitting that you don't have all the answers can be a good sign.)

## Dare to Ask For Specifics

Whenever your prospective Dominant makes a generic statement, try to narrow the focus down to something specific. Asking for names, dates, people, places, and rational reasons for the things he's done can be extremely informative. After all, it's relatively easy to bluff your way through a generic discussion. It becomes exponentially more difficult to bluff your way through a minefield of specifics, especially if those specifics can be fact-checked. Google is your friend.

Here are some examples of how you can get more *specifics* in the course of your interview:

So, you were a member of a BDSM munch group in Seattle? That's fascinating! What was it called?

You know Shibari? Cool! Which type of rope harness do you employ the most?

You regularly go to a public dungeon? Which one?

Encouraging him to offer more than bland generalities is a valuable skill that can serve you well in plenty of other areas in your life, as well. You'll be amazed at how effective it can be against anyone who pretends to have knowledge that he lacks in reality.

## Get a Second Opinion

Any Dominant who is worth your time will typically have no problem with meeting your friends, whether it is in an online chat or face-to-face. If he does, something probably isn't right. If he refuses to interact in any way with your current circle of friends *now*, what do you think will happen *after* you're collared? Attempting to cut you off from your friends or family is almost always a sign of an exploitative or predatory relationship.

Just tell him, "I'd love to introduce you to my friends!" If you're lucky, you have friends who are in the lifestyle, skilled at conducting interviews, or highly intuitive when they meet new people. If you're *not* that lucky and none of your friends are great interrogators, just ask someone whose judgment you trust to meet your prospective Dom.

When you *do,* trust their intuition. I can't even begin to count the number of times that I've been asked to do this very thing for a friend, only to have my opinion ignored because it didn't agree with what she wanted to hear. Then, weeks later, she'll grouse about how she should've listened to her friends' warnings.

## Don't Stop Wondering

Just because your initial interview may have gone well, that doesn't mean you should now check your curiosity at the door as you continue to explore a potential relationship with this Dominant.

Curiosity is a good thing, as is a good memory. Make it a point to remember the things he tells you. You can't serve your Dominant well unless you know your Dominant well, so this is entirely within the scope of what every good submissive should be doing *anyway*. Until you have learned enough about your prospective Dominant that you would trust your life to him, you have not learned enough about him. In fact, you just *may* end up trusting your life to this person at some point in the future.

Each of the tips I've given you thus far is designed to assist you in getting the information that you'll need in order to make an informed decision about whether your prospective Dominant is worthy of your submission.

We frequently hear talk of the so-called *Gift of Submission*, but, in reality, I'm not so sure it qualifies as a gift by the strictest definition of the word. After all, a gift is something that is offered with no expectation of anything received in return.

When it comes to D/s relationships, you typically do expect something in return for your submission. You expect to be treated with respect and with love. You expect to be able to trust that your partner will not harm you or those you care about. You expect that he does what he does because it is good for you, rather than just good for him. You expect to be told the truth and you should have an expectation that he is who and what he says he is.

These are not unrealistic expectations and you should never allow anyone to try and convince you that they are. You deserve to find happiness in this lifestyle and you should expect to find the kind of partner you deserve, but *only* if you're willing to do what is necessary to accomplish that goal. That means asking the right questions.

# Chapter 2: Before You Meet

Much of this book is written on the assumption that most people will become acquainted with their prospective partners online or by telephone before meeting face-to-face. Twenty years ago, this was typically not the case, but it is *now* a fact of life for the great majority of people in the BDSM lifestyle. If you don't use the internet and don't text or message, you needn't feel that you must skip this chapter. Just address the topics covered in this chapter at your earliest opportunity as you get further acquainted with your prospective Dominant.

Remember, it isn't always enough to simply ask the right questions. It's also imperative that you ask the right questions at the right time. Timing is everything. To that end, I have made some effort to categorize the suggested questions in this book into sections based upon when and where they will do you the most good.

Hopefully, you'll ask the questions designed to keep you safe and alive before you actually meet him in real life. It won't help to get clarification on what a collar symbolizes to your prospective Dominant after he has already padlocked it around your neck. Similarly, questions designed to enhance your relationship probably won't be useful to you before you're in a relationship.

So, *yes*. Timing really *is* everything.

This section focuses on the questions that you should be asking your prospective Dominant before you decide to meet face-to-face. These questions are intended to accomplish three things: (1) Save you the time, trouble and expense of meeting someone who later turns out to be one of those creeps that you would normally scoot away from on a bus stop bench, (2) Save you from the emotional investment, gut-wrenching *pain,* and crippling social embarrassment of falling for an imposter, and (3) Keep you alive and safe from harm. I have seen *all* of these things happen to friends again and again because they trusted their feelings, instead of trusting a sound strategy for finding the right lifestyle partner.

## New Relationship Energy (NRE)

You're probably familiar with the term *New Relationship Energy* (NRE) and perhaps even found yourself enveloped in it at one point or another in your lifetime. NRE is that wonderful, giddy feeling you get in the initial phases of any budding relationship. The intensity of NRE can surprise even the most jaded individuals and it can be extremely easy to start believing that this intense, amazing feeling is a sign or omen of the perfection and rightness of the situation. It *isn't.*

Let me say this again, with proper emphasis: ***It is not.***

New Relationship Energy is a result of neurochemical substance called dopamine which makes you feel euphoric and happy. When you start to fall in love, dopamine is released by your brain into your system. Dopamine is the reason you can stay up all night chatting with your partner on the phone or dancing the night away on a secluded beach. It's what makes you feel sexy, smart, appreciated, bold, energetic, and willing to take risks you otherwise would have avoided. It's also why you stop relying on common sense, believe the unbelievable, and do incredibly stupid things while in its grip.

Dopamine has its good side, too. Aside from its obvious euphoric effects, dopamine is thought to be a significant factor in how Parkinson's disease, schizophrenia, ADHD, and many other mental disorders affect our well-being. You've heard that love cures all? Well, it doesn't cure everything, but it just may have some basis in truth. When you fall in love, the dopamine released into your system as a result of a new relationship can reduce the impact of certain mental and physical disorders.

Consider this little-known fact: Many anti-psychotic drug treatments work by altering the dopamine levels in your system. Here's the part that should give you pause. Taking anti-psychotic medications every day can give you a lifetime of relief from your mental disorders but eventually, new relationship energy wears off. When it does, the euphoria fades and the positive effects of your natural anti-psychotic neurochemicals fade as well.

Now you're back to being the person you were before that whole giddy, floating on cloud nine thing. Suddenly, the rational side of your brain starts working again and an awful lot of those answers that he gave you that seemed to make sense just a few months ago just *don't* any more.

*That's* why you need this book.

Dopamine *giveth* and it *taketh* away, but this book can keep you out of trouble for as long as you're willing to keep it and use it.

**Question #1:** Why are you interested in me?

**Follow-up questions:**

What is it about me that interests you?

Was there something on my personal profile that stood out or caught your eye?

What do you *think* you know about me?

Is there something more about me that you would like to know?

**Why it's important:**

It truly pains me to have to say this about my own gender, but here it is, in a nutshell: Sometimes, he isn't really interested in you as an individual. Sometimes, it's simply that he has approached fifty people today, and you are the only one who has responded to his approach in a friendly way. He'll never admit to this, of course, and that's why you ask follow-up questions to find out if he has even bothered to look at your profile or learn anything at *all* about you before approaching you.

**How to interpret the answer:**

You're not fishing for compliments or flattery here, so don't be swayed by it when he starts to lay it on thick. Press for specifics. If he says he loves your eyes, ask him if he even has a clue what color they are. If he says he loves your body-type, ask him which body type he's referring to. If he says he lives in the same town, ask him for the name of the town or to describe some of his favorite hangouts there. Nine times out of ten, you'll discover that he hasn't even bothered to read your profile, and hasn't even glanced at your photos until *after* you started questioning him. Very often, a phony will tell you that he's local to you, even when he has no idea where you live.

## What you should do about it:

Learn to recognize their use of this fishing strategy. They typically cast a very wide net, hoping to pull in someone - *anyone* - who doesn't realize that they are just one of dozens of submissives being flattered and charmed that day. They do this because many new submissives are naive and vulnerable, and are anxious to find a partner. They do this because it fuels their sex and power fantasies and provides them with free real-life porn. It is an entertaining game to them, nothing more.

In the final analysis, he does what he does because it works for him. Learn to recognize when he is bluffing, and how to call his bluff.

## My Two Cents:

"Oh look, Master!" exclaimed Kitten, "I just got a message from a local Dom who goes to the same college I do!"

Kitten was always interested in making new BDSM lifestyle friends, so her excitement wasn't at all unusual. She usually kept me informed about her circle of friends and trusted my judgment regarding how to handle them. I was a little intrigued about this particular new friend.

"What's his name?" I asked, thinking that I might know him from my dealings with the local kink community.

"Hmmm," she replied, searching her laptop screen to find it. "Vadish Desai."

"Sounds Indian to me," I said. "And he says that he's local and goes to your college?"

She nodded. "Yes, Master." and showed me the chat on her laptop screen.

I grinned, because I'd noticed something that she'd missed. He had carefully avoided ever mentioning the name of the college or the town. "Ask him for the names of his favorite professors there, Kitten."

She looked a little perplexed. "Ummm... *Why?*"

"Just do it." I replied.

She did, and it soon became apparent that she wasn't going to get any sort of a timely answer. Eventually, she did get another message, but it wasn't the response she was expecting.

"Master," she giggled, "*Now*, he is asking me to send him a picture of myself!"

*What a surprise*, I thought, grinning. "Tell him you'll do even better than that. Tell him that you want to meet him, and that you'll be at the local Denny's restaurant in thirty minutes. Tell him you'll wait for him up front at the hostess station and that you'll be wearing a black skirt with no panties, a red blouse, and a flower in your hair."

"Whaaaaaat?!?" she squeaked, incredulously. "Why in the world would I tell him *that*, Master?"

I laughed, "Because if he is real, he'll make it a point to tell you that there *is* no Denny's restaurant in this town."

**Question #2:** How would you like to be addressed?

**Follow-up questions:**

Why do you like to be addressed in that manner?

Who else addresses you in this fashion?

Why does Person#1 call you that, when Person#2 does not?

**Why it's important:**

First, it's important because you want to avoid inadvertently disrespecting your prospective Dominant during the interview. Second, it's important because if your interview process is successful, you just may have to get used to addressing him in that fashion. Third, his *reasoning* for his preference will often tell you a lot about him.

**How to interpret his answer:**

If he likes to be addressed as *Sir*, even by strangers, there's nothing particularly odd or megalomaniacal about that. In the southern states, a lot of people will call even complete strangers Sir. I spent twenty years in the US army calling thousands of people Sir simply as a matter of courtesy. A common rule of thumb in the kink community has always been, if you don't know how someone wants to be addressed, simply start with Sir or Ma'am. They will immediately inform you if it bothers them and instruct you on how they prefer to be addressed. If, on the other hand, someone demands that strangers call him Master, Daddy, or *Grand Imperial Poohbah*, that might just turn out to be a yellow flag.

**What you should do about it:**

Render the appropriate level of respect to others in the lifestyle, and don't get too caught up in the notion that you shouldn't observe lifestyle customs, courtesies, and protocols just because someone hasn't yet "earned" your respect. Remember, you probably want to be treated with respect too. What, exactly, have *you* done to earn *his* respect?

**My Two Cents:**

Just in case you didn't know this about me, I'm half Asian. In much of Asia, it is considered extremely rude to address someone by their name. I know, I know. Seems rather silly, doesn't it? Why give someone a name, if you can't actually call them by it?

This custom is the reason why you hear Asians commonly referring to others by familial appellations like Brother, Sister, Uncle, or Grandfather even if they are not actually *related* to those people. Even calling someone "Old Man" or "Old Woman" is often considered more polite than addressing them by their first name! That's the culture I grew up in.

I also spent over twenty years in the military, where *Sir* and *Ma'am* are a simple matter of courtesy, whether you know the individual or not; whether he or she has earned your respect or not.

I am often asked how I like to be addressed, and my answer is usually, "I prefer to be called *Sir* by my friends and associates. I don't demand it, it is simply my preference. My collared submissives call me *Master*. I suppose you can call me whatever you please, as long as it isn't Master, and as long as it isn't disrespectful. Frankly, if you do not feel that I deserve to be addressed as I wish, then by that same standard, you've not earned enough respect to be addressed as you wish, either. So, maybe I'll just call you *Ralph* from now on."

**Question #3:** Is there a certain way you would like to address me, once we are in a relationship?

**Follow-up questions:**

Why would you want to call me that?

Have you always called your relationship partners that?

What kinds of pet names or endearments do you like in general?

Which ones tend to rub you the wrong way?

**Why it's important:**

It's important because this can sometimes be one of those things that completely blindsides you when you least expect it because you never bothered to find out that he likes to refer to his subs as *slut*, *whore*, *piggy*, or as his *little fuck-toy*.

**How to interpret his answer:**

Take what he tells in response to this question at face value. Don't ever assume that he isn't being serious about it, even if it seems like he may be joking or teasing when he says it. In practically every joke, there is always a kernel of truth to be found.

**What you should do about it:**

If you aren't going to like being called whatever it is he likes to call his submissives, there's no time like the present to speak up.

**My Two Cents:**

"Would you ever call me your little cum slut or your fuck-toy?"

I must admit, the question caught me a little by surprise. I was being interviewed by a prospective submissive named Jenny and up to that point her questions had been pretty straightforward and relatively easy to answer. Now this.

"I highly doubt it," I replied. "I hold my submissives in high regard and I really do treasure their gift of submission. I *cherish* my subs; I don't enjoy degrading or humiliating them."

"Too bad," she groused, "I really wanted to be called your *little cum slut* and *fuck toy*."

**Question #4:** Are you married or currently in a committed relationship?

**Follow-up questions:**

What's your definition of a committed relationship?

Have you been married before? If so, what happened?

Are you divorced or separated?

What are your views on marriage?

**Why it's important:**

You may or may not have specific goals in mind when it comes to marriage or committed relationships, but you can be sure that if the two of you have completely different objectives in this regard, there's a very high probability that it is going to turn into a serious train wreck.

**How to interpret his answer:**

Whatever the response to your question about his views on marriage, be sure to believe it. It's extremely rare for someone to change their thinking on something like whether or not they believe in marriage.

**What you should do about it:**

Resist at all costs the urge to gloss over or ignore the answers to this set of questions just because you don't happen to like them. If *you* want a marriage and your prospective Mr. Right doesn't believe in marriage, that makes him Mr. Wrong.

**My Two Cents:**

I met Jade almost ten years ago in a dungeon, but not the BDSM kind. It was an online virtual dungeon in a massively multiplayer online role-playing game called *Ultima Online*. Yes, that's how we courted - in a geeky swords and sorcery game.

One day, after an epic Sunday afternoon of monster-slaying and puzzle solving, we found ourselves strolling virtually through a beautiful, secret underground garden. I sat on a log, thinking this would be a nice place to chat. Suddenly and quite unexpectedly, her avatar was in my lap. I guess I'll never know if it was on purpose or simply the result of a mistaken mouse-click, but neither of us made a move to extricate ourselves from this unexpected bit of coziness.

"Whoops!" she said. "Hmm. I seem to be in your lap, Sir."

I grinned. "Yes, you *do* seem to be in my lap. Not that I'm complaining, mind you!"

She chuckled and said, "Well, how bad could it be? It's not like you're *married*, or anything, right?"

Now, it was my turn to chuckle, since I was, indeed married at the time. I said, "Actually, I am married. Happily married, in fact, and it is highly unlikely that anyone would ever be able to take me away from her."

Years later, long after accepting my collar, Jade told me that *that* was the moment she knew. Those were the words that convinced her that she wanted to be mine.

**Question #5:** How far would you be willing to go to prove to me that you're not full of crap?

**Follow-up questions:**

Why or why not?

**Why it's important:**

This question should be posed as a hypothetical, but sooner or later, you may have to ask your prospective Dominant to put up or shut up, particularly if there are gaping holes in his story. Knowing ahead of time just how hard you can push will definitely be important.

**How to interpret his answer:**

There really is only *one* practical, acceptable answer to this question, and it is, "I will take whatever *reasonable* steps may be necessary to demonstrate to you that I am telling you the truth."

The other two possibilities, not nearly as practical or acceptable are: (1) "Either you believe me, or you don't. Take it or leave it." and from the other end of the spectrum, (2) "I will do anything!" Either of those responses should earn at *least* a yellow flag.

**What you should do about it:**

File his answer away for future reference. Sooner or later, it is going to come in handy. Oh, and never forget that just because something sounds unbelievable, that doesn't necessarily mean it's a lie.

**My Two Cents:**

I've been on the receiving end of that *"you're full of crap"* thing before. It's no fun, I can tell you that.

If you've read any of my other books, you already know that I've lived a pretty unusual life, done some incredible things, and known tons of crazy people. That doesn't necessarily make it untrue; it just makes some of it very hard to believe.

I *get* it. I really *do*.

A few years ago, I was casually being considered by a feisty submissive named Janine, a young woman who was pretty adept at asking great questions. Over the course of several weeks, she succeeded in tactfully asking me dozens of probing questions, all of which were effective in getting me to talk about my rather peculiar life. The only problem was, she could barely conceal her growing skepticism and rather obvious contempt for my answers.

One evening, as we participated in a group discussion with friends, the conversation turned to pet peeves. Each person volunteered an amusing pet peeve, such as leaving the toilet seat up, plus-sized women in spandex pants, or people who grind their teeth in their sleep. I'm not sure what may have been on my mind at the time, but when my turn came, I said, "My pet peeve is people who stand around with their thumbs up their butts while someone is *dying*, right there, in front of them."

There was a moment of stunned silence in the room, during which Janine apparently decided she'd heard just about enough of my bullcrap. She snarkily remarked, "Oh, and I suppose that sort of thing happens around you all the time, eh? I don't suppose you can offer us a recent example of what you mean, *can* you?"

If you know me at all, then you know this one defining thing about me: I never bluff. If you think I'm bluffing and decide to call my bluff, you're going to be in for a rude surprise. This instance was no exception.

I told the story of how, less than a year earlier, I'd been one of the first to arrive on the scene of a serious automobile accident on the outskirts of town. There had been three people in the car. The driver was a middle-aged woman and in the passenger seat was her twelve-year old daughter. Her ten-year old son had been sitting on the driver's side of the back seat. As they passed through a highway intersection, their car was broadsided at 60 mph by a driver who ran a red light. The impact crushed the driver's side back end of the car and threw the wreckage onto a nearby embankment.

When I arrived, there were three men standing there, just looking at the wreckage. It took me a moment to realize that there were still people in the wreckage of the car. I told the three men to help me get the people out of the car, and they grudgingly did so.

The mother and daughter were relatively unhurt and needed to be treated for shock, but the little boy in the back seat was broken up pretty badly. I have some Army combat medical training, so I checked his pulse and respiration. He had a weak pulse and no respiration. I realized that he was probably going to die if he didn't get CPR immediately, so I began chest compressions and rescue breathing.

His mother, still in a severe state of shock and huddled under a blanket, saw what I was doing and began screaming and pointing at me. "Somebody stop him!" she cried out hysterically, "Don't touch my son! You're going to hurt him! Somebody *stop that man!*"

The same three men who earlier had to be prodded to pull these people out of the smoking car wreckage were *now* suddenly full of initiative. They pounced on me and dragged me off the little boy while I was in mid-breath, trying to force precious air into his lungs. The three of them held me forcefully, even as I begged them to let me save his life. For the next three minutes, we stood there as the life just drained out of that little boy's body. A few minutes later, an ambulance arrived and only then did the men release their grip on me. The paramedics pronounced him dead on the scene.

Disgusted and angry, I got back into my car and drove away. Every few weeks, I have to drive through that intersection and I see a small cross with his name on it that his parents have erected on the very spot where he died. His name was *Chance*. I'm done being angry about it, but it still makes me sad to think about it.

At the conclusion of my story, Janine was unable to contain her skepticism any longer. With a look of pure contempt on her face, she exclaimed, "What a bunch of shit! Do you think we're all morons? Do you seriously expect us to believe that the mother and daughter didn't have a scratch on them, but the boy in the back seat was killed? You expect us to believe people stood around and did nothing? And really... who in the world names their kid *Chance?* Surely, you could have come up with a better name than that! You must take us all for fools!"

It takes a *lot* to make me angry. And how does one know that I am angry? I get quiet and methodical. I do whatever it takes to make you *wish* I were loud and not in control of my emotions. I showed Janine a small collection of newspaper clippings about the accident, some photographs of the cross at the intersection, and a copy of Chance's obituary. Then, I told her exactly what I thought of any smarmy little know-it-all who would stoop to puffing herself up by ridiculing the unnecessary death of a helpless little boy. She was sobbing by the time I was done with her and, frankly, I was glad of it.

The interview was now *over*.

**Question #6:** How long have you been in the BDSM lifestyle?

**Follow-up questions:**

What's your definition of "being in the BDSM lifestyle?"

What makes it a "lifestyle" for you?

What parts of your life are impacted by your BDSM interests and activities?

**Why it's important:**

Some people have a pretty broad definition of what it means to be "in the lifestyle." Some may feel that simply having an interest in it or reading books about it should qualify. Others think that just because they tried something kinky in bed once ten years ago, that that should be counted as ten years of experience in the lifestyle! Needless to say, this is one of those crucial questions where you have to probe for specifics if you want anything useful.

**How to interpret his answer:**

There are an infinite number of ways you can dissect your prospective Dominant's answer to this question, but *do* remember this: It's called a lifestyle because it impacts significant portions of your life. If a person's sum of experience consists solely of a few kinky bedroom activities, I would be hesitant about making that the basis of an entire *lifestyle*. By the same logic, a lot of people would have to consider themselves to be a part of the *blow-job* lifestyle or the *missionary position* lifestyle.

**What you should do about it:**

Take his responses with a grain of salt. Get specifics and decide whether he is inflating his resume. Then, make up your own mind about how important it is to you.

**My Two Cents:**

William was visiting our BDSM chat room for the very first time and, as a result, members of the group were enthusiastically peppering him with a ton of questions. Eventually, one of the subs in the room asked him, "How long have you been in the BDSM lifestyle?"

"Fifteen years," he replied, without a moment's hesitation.

Very impressive, I thought. Even so, the skeptic in me simply wasn't content to blindly accept it at face value. I dug a little deeper into his personal profile and even Googled his username. The guy certainly wasn't hiding, that was for sure. His very unique username was all over the internet... and he was just twenty one years old. Imagine that!

He was still regaling the group with tales of his Domly Domminess when I asked him if he was really just twenty-one years old. He was momentarily taken aback, surprised that someone had bothered to check up on him, but then he admitted that he was, indeed, twenty one. It's entirely possible that, at this particular point in the conversation, he simply hadn't yet done the math.

"So," I continued, "Are you seriously trying to tell us that you've been in the BDSM lifestyle since you were *six years old?*"

"Yes," he answered, "I was taken captive as a slave when I was six years old. It was only after I killed my Mistress at age eight that I was able to escape and become a full-fledged Dominant."

Boot. Block. *Next!*

**Question #7:** How long have you been a Dominant?

**Follow-up questions:**

How do you know you are a Dominant?

What makes you think you are a Dominant?

How do you feel about being a Dominant?

**Why it's important:**

He may or may not actually *be* a Dominant. If he isn't, that could be the result of an intentional deception or it could be a matter of self-delusion. His responses to these questions may give you the clues you need to figure out just what is going on there.

**How to interpret his answer:**

When this question is posed in an interview, it *seems* like a perfectly simple, easy to answer question. It is *not*. For any true Dominant, this question is going to be a real challenge. Your analysis of his answers will probably be equally difficult. Imagine having to answer a question like, "How do you feel about being a woman?" The range of responses could range from flippant and superficial to deeply thoughtful and philosophically profound. If his response is given proper consideration, the answer should be complex, yet enlightening.

**What you should do about it:**

Ponder his responses over a period of time. Write them down, if necessary, so you can refer back to them at a later date as new ideas occur to you, or as you learn more about your prospective Dominant. Don't rest until *you* can distill his reasoning down to a single sentence that encapsulates what you know about him as a Dominant and makes perfect sense to you. Then, and *only* then, are you done with this question.

**My Two Cents:**

I have posted my own response to this particular question in various writings, forums, and memes but here it is again for anyone who may have missed it.

For *me*, being a Dominant isn't about telling people what to do, or using it as a way to mask your own insecurities. It's simply about being the master of your own destiny; controlling your environment, and being so damn good at it that people want to be part of your environment, and share your destiny.

**Question #8:** How did you come to realize that you were a Dominant?

**Follow-up questions:**

Did you start out as a submissive or switch?

Do you believe Dominants are made or born?

If you trained to be a Dominant, how did you do that?

Did you have a mentor or guide in becoming a Dominant?

**Why it's important:**

The "nature versus nurture" argument has been around since time immemorial, when it comes to child-rearing and genetics, but it's a relatively new controversy to the BDSM lifestyle. Some people believe that "real" Dominants are born, not trained. Some believe that you can't be a good Dominant unless you have experience what it is like to be a submissive, first. Still others believe that practically *anyone* can become a Dominant with the right guidance and training. What do *you* believe?

**How to interpret his answer:**

Obviously, there is no right or wrong response to this question however, assuming you have strong beliefs one way or another regarding whether Doms are born or trained, you might want to ensure that your beliefs on this are compatible.

**What you should do about it:**

If you happen to believe that anyone can be trained to be a Dominant, then you should seek out a Dominant who has sufficient training. If, on the other hand, you are a true believer in the notion that some people are natural born Dominants, then you should seek out someone who *was*. If you honestly don't know what you think, you should decide to decide. This is an issue that will come up again and again for you, for as long as you are in this lifestyle.

**My Two Cents:**

My personal belief, when it comes to the question of whether Doms are born or made, happens to lean heavily in the direction of genetics. I am a Dominant, my father is dominant, and my father's father was likewise extremely dominant.

Even so, I recognize that genetics can only do *so* much. A person's DNA may help to determine his potential, but the tools, resources, and training that he gets in life also help to flesh out the person he was meant to be. I don't doubt for a moment that my twenty years in the military helped me to *hone* my leadership, mentoring, and communication skills.

How different a Dominant I would have been, if I'd taken another career path, is *anyone's* guess.

**Question #9:** How old are you?

**Follow-up questions:**

No, *really*. How old are you?

**Why it's important:**

It's only important if you feel that a significant age gap between you and your relationship partner could be a *deal-breaker*.

**How to interpret his answer:**

Compare his answer to his observed behavior and apparent maturity level.

**What you should do about it:**

Record it or remember it for future reference. Eventually, you'll get a chance to verify his age. It may or may not matter to you, but do it anyway. You just never know when and how it will turn out to be useful or necessary.

**My Two Cents:**

The interview had been going quite well, right up until we got to the part where she asked me how old I was.

"I don't discuss my age," I said, tersely.

Alice seemed undeterred by my effort to sidestep the question. "You can tell *me*," she said. "I don't care how old you are. Age is just a number, as far as I am concerned."

I raised an eyebrow at her, and replied, "If you *really* don't care, and if age is just a number, then why is it so important for you to know how old I am?"

"I'm just curious," she replied, sassily.

I rolled my eyes and countered, "Be curious about something else."

Alice couldn't let go of it, though. "Seriously, Sir. You can tell *me*. Why is it such a big deal? You know how old I am. Why won't you just tell me how old you are? I really don't *care* how old you are, I just want to *know*, that's all!"

I sighed in exasperation. "You just don't get it, do you? This isn't about whether or not *you* care about how old I am. The fact at the heart of this matter is *I* care about how old I am. I'm getting older, and I don't particularly *like* it. My age is no big *secret*, but I simply don't like thinking about it, I don't like talking about it, and I definitely don't like arguing about it, so just drop it. Have I made myself clear on this?"

Alice nodded silently and waited about an hour before asking me again.

**Question #10:** What sort of work do you do?

**Follow-up questions:**

Do you enjoy it?

What is it about that sort of work that you enjoy/dislike?

How long have you been in this line of work?

**Why it's important:**

Knowing what sort of work a person does can give you a great deal of insight into how he thinks, what his priorities are, and what skills he has. Knowing how long he's been at this job can help you ascertain his career stability, momentum, and *"stick-to-itiveness."* And *yes*, I just made that word up.

**How to interpret his answer:**

What does his work tell you about how he thinks or how he conducts himself? Does he work with ideas, or with his hands? Is he highly skilled or not? Are his skills valuable, or not? Is he competitive? View his work through these prisms.

**What you should do about it:**

If you are the sort of person who categorizes certain types of work as being undesirable, low-paying, or low-status jobs then you should probably seek a partner who isn't going to be happy staying in one of those kinds of jobs. If you prefer the cerebral type, seek a partner who deals in ideas. If you prefer a partner who works with his hands, his line of work can be a guidepost for you. And obviously, his position in the hierarchy of an organization can tell you quite a bit about his competitive or dominant nature. A true Dominant who is competent, competitive, and alpha outside of the bedroom doesn't stay at the bottom of any corporate ladder for very long.

**My Two Cents:**

I've never been particularly handy at building or fixing things with my own two hands. When I was sixteen, I realized I would never be good at auto repair when I discovered that laying on my back and looking up into the engine compartment of a car made me dizzy and nauseous. Hopefully, I'll never have to paint my own *ceiling* because, even now, the simple act of changing a light bulb in a ceiling fixture makes me want to *spew*.

How many Dominants does it take to change a light bulb in *my* house? *None*.

On the other hand, twenty years of military service has taught me a boatload of combat and survival skills. Give me a multi-tool and some paracord and I'm like a geeky *MacGyver on crack*.

A prospective submissive named Tina once asked me what kind of work I did. I explained that I've been a waiter, bartender, restaurant manager, soldier, stock trader, magazine publisher, banker, paramilitary equipment retailer, advertising executive, freelance writer, website designer, kink-toy retailer, small business consultant, and even sold blow-up sex dolls as I worked my way through college.

"Ah, *I see,*" she said, "A Jack-of-all-trades! Well, is there anything you *haven't* done or won't do?"

I laughed and replied, "I don't paint ceilings or change light bulbs."

**Question #11:** Where do you live?

**Follow-up questions:**

What city? What *part* of the city?

How long have you lived there?

Why did you choose to live there or to stay there?

Ask about nearby landmarks or culturally unique features of that city.

**Why it's important:**

This is one of those questions that typically isn't important, until you find out that your new online friend also happens to be your next door neighbor. Then, it gets a whole lot more important, really fast. It may also become important if you decide that you want to meet face-to-face or in the eventuality that some day the two of you will have to start thinking about where you may want to live together as a committed couple.

**How to interpret his answer:**

Watch for indications that he may not actually be where he *says* he is. Ask for plenty of specifics and compare the information he gives you with what you already know about the place or can readily look up.

**What you should do about it:**

If it turns out that he isn't being truthful, tactfully discuss it with him to learn why he may have felt it was necessary and appropriate to be deceptive about it. Otherwise, compare his preference and reasoning with your own as it pertains to where you each would like to live, long term.

**My Two Cents:**

Hasi was a single 26-year old Japanese girl who worked as a bar manager in Tokyo, Japan to support her 10 year old daughter. We chatted online almost daily and after a few months she began asking me a *lot* of probing questions. Normally, that wouldn't be a problem, but I kept getting the feeling that something wasn't quite right about Hasi, so I kept her at arm's length.

One day, she was worried about possibly moving from Tokyo to Okinawa, which was almost 1300 miles away and a place where she supposedly didn't know anyone. The following week, she was already there, just like *magic*. Within a few days, she suddenly had an address book full of close friends in Okinawa. She was even spending time at the hospital bedside of her "childhood best friend" in Okinawa, who was dying of cancer. All very suspicious, but it wasn't my circus; not my monkey.

Then, she did something bizarre, even for *her*. She taught her ten-year old daughter how to chat online and brought her into our BDSM chat room to introduce her to the members of the group! We politely told her that it was inappropriate to have her child in the room and asked her to leave. As a result, most of us became convinced at that time that her daughter didn't actually exist at *all*. It was beginning to look like a mental illness or some kind of bizarre multi-character role-play masquerading as real-life.

We became even more convinced that it was a grand deception when, just a few days later during a discussion about drinking, Hasi said she was drinking some tequila shots at that very moment. A quick check of a world-clock told me that it was seven o'clock A.M. tomorrow morning (which was a Wednesday) in Okinawa. I asked myself, what single mom of a ten-year old girl does tequila shots at *seven in the morning*, on a school day?

Even so, I was still willing to ignore her deception, figuring it was none of my business. But then Hasi began stalking with a close female friend of mine and pressured her for things like cyber-sex and nude photos. Consequently, I *made* it my business.

I tracked Hasi's IP address and learned that she wasn't in Okinawa, at all! She was in Kansas City, Missouri. I tracked her profile photos and learned that they, too, were phony. They'd been stolen from a pretty Chinese Hankook Racing model who lived in Hong Kong.

Finally, I had my friend send Hasi a photo with a stealthy little bit of programming code that helped us to identify Hasi as a married 47-year old male Pakistani grocery store owner in Kansas City. His "thing" was impersonating a kawaii (*cute*) bisexual Japanese girl so he could more easily engage in cyber-sex with young, naive girls.

It's ironic that, in the end, he was tripped up by the simplest of questions: *Where do you live?*

**Question #12:** Are you financially secure?

**Follow-up questions:**

Does it make you uncomfortable to discuss this subject with me?

Do you depend on someone else, such as a parent, spouse, or government entitlements for financial support?

Are you paying child support?

Are you paying alimony to an ex-spouse?

Have I overstepped any boundaries by bring this subject up?

**Why it's important:**

The question itself isn't anywhere near as important as his reaction to it will be.

**How to interpret his answer:**

Frankly, this is one of those questions that come perilously close to exceeding the limits of good manners. At this point in the process, how much money he makes or has in the bank *really* isn't any of your business. Even so, his reaction to the question will tell you a lot about him. And who knows, he may even give you an honest answer, though that is an admittedly unlikely scenario.

**What you should do about it:**

Don't get your panties in a bunch if he tells you that it's none of your damn business. After all, it really isn't. But then, you already *know* that. You should neither be surprised nor offended if he gives you an evasive or less than honest answer. In fact, you should probably treat any answer he gives you as less than honest. Just take it in stride, accept it as one more piece of the puzzle that you're assembling, and move on to the next question.

**My Two Cents:**

Lisa was cautioning me about her new friend, Cathy. "Daddy, you're really going to have to keep an eye on that one, if and when you ever do get a chance to meet her."

I laughed out loud and asked, "Why do you think so, babygirl?"

"Because," she said, "as soon as she found out that my Daddy was a best-selling BDSM author, the first thing out of her mouth was, Wow! He must be making money hand-over-fist! Will you introduce me to him?"

I laughed again, harder this time. "Did you tell her she's going to have to buy me lunch if she wants to meet me? I'm a starving writer, after all."

She giggled at the idea and replied, "You know I would never discuss your finances with some stranger, Daddy!"

Yes, I *did* know that and was exceedingly glad. I've not yet had the pleasure of meeting the woman in question, whom Lisa now refers to as "that subbie-gold-digger," but when I do, I better get at least a *sandwich* out of the deal.

**Question #13:** Which do you prefer, SSC or RACK?

**Follow-up questions:**

Why is that your preference?

**Why it's important:**

It's a simple way to ascertain whether your prospective Dominant is knowledgeable about the BDSM lifestyle in general and lifestyle safety issues in particular.

**How to interpret his answer:**

Either preference is acceptable, as long as he knows what the acronyms stand for. By the way, the acronyms stand for Safe, Sane & Consensual (SSC) and Risk Aware Consensual Kink (RACK). His reasoning for his preference should be considered icing on the cake, but only if it makes any sense at all.

**What you should do about it:**

Treat any attempt to bluff his way through this question as a red flag. Not every effort to bluff or *bullshit you* deserves the red flag treatment, but when it comes to your personal safety, that's another matter, entirely.

**My Two Cents:**

Personally, I never much liked the whole SSC concept. After all, who's to say what's safe and what isn't? I'm a former Army paratrooper. Is jumping out of a perfectly good airplane, even with a parachute, a safe thing to do? I'm guessing there might be some debate amongst my friends and readers about that.

The issue of what should be considered sane is similarly problematic. One man's sanity is another man's crazy, and vice versa. The BDSM lifestyle is full of activities that are commonplace and even trendy today that would have been called insane just twenty years ago.

One would at least think that the word *consensual* still means what it always has always meant, but *au contraire!* Just try dipping your toe into any discussion about consensual non-consent, and you'll see what I mean.

Frankly, I'm much more comfortable with the RACK principles. Nothing is ever going to be entirely safe and no one really knows what sane means anymore. But, hopefully, we can all agree that good decisions regarding BDSM play can only be made if you are fully aware of the *risks* involved.

The only way to do *that* is to *educate* yourselves.

**Question #14:** Do you belong to any lifestyle-related organizations or munch groups?

**Follow-up questions:**

If not, why not?

What are the names of the groups you belong to?

How would you feel about me joining that group, too?

**Why it's important:**

This question touches on several important issues on a variety of levels. It helps you to gauge his social skills, the depth of his personal network, his lifestyle experiences and knowledge, and perhaps even his integrity.

**How to interpret his answer:**

Pay close attention to his response. Make an attempt to verify what he says regarding his group activities.

**What you should do about it:**

Talk to other members of the group in question, if at all possible. Consider attending future group functions if it is practical for you to do so. If he is averse to participating in any group activities you should consider that a yellow flag worthy of some follow-up.

**My Two Cents:**

"I don't belong to the local BDSM group," huffed Anthony. "All of the people in that group are posers and phonies. I refuse to have anything to do with them."

Julia was on her first date with Anthony, a prospective Dominant who'd met her for dinner at a local seafood restaurant. They'd barely made it to the salad course when she became irritated by his response to a question about the local kinksters group. She pressed him further. "Who, in particular, are you talking about? I mean, I happen to *know* some of those people in the group. They are good people. Which are the posers and phonies, in your opinion?"

Anthony bristled at being put on the spot and replied, "All of them! Not a damn one of them knows what they're doing. If you want a *real* Master, you need to stop hanging out with that group of losers, and just let me teach you whatever you need to know."

Julia was instantly livid. "You know what, *Mr. Full-of-Yourself?* I've been a member of that group for two years and those people are the nicest, most knowledgeable people you'll ever meet. For you to say that all 240 members of the group are posers and phonies just told me everything I need to know about *you!* You're a pathetic loser, lurking around the fringes of the local community like some kind of a hyena, hoping to pick off a member of the herd that is weak, confused, or isolated. I'm guessing the *real* reason you don't participate in group activities is because *they* won't have anything to do with *you!"*

A few days later, after discussing the experience over coffee with some members of the group's managing committee, Julia learned that she'd guessed right. Anthony had long ago been banned from the group's activities for repeated instances of inappropriate behavior.

**Question #15:** Do you frequent BDSM chat rooms or discussion groups?

**Follow-up questions:**

Do you frequent any lifestyle-related websites or forums?

Are you a member of Fetlife?

Do you have a profile on any lifestyle-related dating sites?

**Why it's important:**

First, the more people he interacts with, the easier it is to learn if he is consistently the same person across the board. Second, some of these other forums may give you a base-line for comparison. Third, you may be able to learn interesting and useful things about him from the profiles on these other web sites.

**How to interpret his answer:**

It's highly unlikely that the place where you met him is the first and only place he frequents. If he claims that it is, he may be telling you the truth, but that is also an indicator that he may be very *new* at all of this.

**What you should do about it:**

Make some effort to check out his profiles on the other web sites. If he claims that he has never visited *any* BDSM related web site, take that assertion with a huge grain of salt. Google his username, just to see what pops up. If you do not have a Fetlife.com profile, I highly recommend that you establish one.

**My Two Cents:**

Mr. Twitchy was a Dominant who was a Fetlife friend of a female submissive in my local BDSM munch group. He never attended any of our local munches or parties and he never socialized with anyone we knew or, for that matter, with males at *all*. Apparently, his modus operandi consisted solely of randomly trolling for women online, and that's how he came to ask my friend out for a date. That, in itself, isn't terribly unusual, but it did make it harder to learn much about him when my friend asked me for help digging into his background.

He claimed he wasn't on any other BDSM dating sites, so we simply *googled his username*. Most people tend to be rather unimaginative when it comes to usernames and so they will typically use the same one everywhere. This makes it pretty easy to do some cross-checking. It's harder if the username is a common one but even then, all you have to do is cross-correlate other factors like age, location, or photographs.

Mr. Twitchy was on several other BDSM dating web sites, but his *other* profiles painted a very different picture of himself than the one he'd presented to my friend. On one site, he described himself as being a foot taller than he was in real-life. On another, he was a submissive instead of a Dominant. On still a third, he was primarily interested in *diaper play* as the diaper *wearer*.

Mr. Twitchy never got the date.

**Question #16:** What are your favorite fetishes?

**Follow-up questions:**

Are they true fetishes, or are you just curious about them?

Have you actually done any of those things?

If not, why not?

Are you secretive about or ashamed of your fetishes?

How important is it to you that your partner shares your fetishes?

Is it a deal-breaker if your prospective partner does not share your fetish?

Has that caused any problems in your prior relationships?

**Why it's important:**

A true fetish is something you don't have much choice about. It's also something that can be overwhelming at times. A kink is one thing, but the true definition of a fetish is that it is something that is *necessary* for your arousal and orgasm. If someone has a diaper fetish, it's not something that they can just put on the back shelf and forget about just because you don't happen to be into diapers, yourself.

**How to interpret his answer:**

Attempt to get your prospect to differentiate between his *kinks* and his *fetishes*.

**What you should do about it:**

Compare his answers with the list of activities that you *are* and are *not* willing to participate in. Think about your *own* kinks and fetishes and ask him how he feels about *those*.

**My Two Cents:**

My list of kinks is long, and I find myself adding to it on a fairly regular basis. My true fetishes, however, hardly constitute a list at all, since I have just a *few*.

The nice thing about having a Fetlife or other fetish community profile is the fact that anyone who may be interested in knowing what your kinks are can simply refer to the web site to see the list. Even more interesting is the ability to click on the name of the fetish or kink and not only learn more about it, but see a list of everyone *else* who happens to be into that kink, as well!

Oddly enough, I've recently learned that I happen to be listed as a fetish on Fetlife.com. I'm guessing that I'm really more of a *kink* than a fetish.

**Question #17:** How many submissives do you have?

Does a submissive have to be collared to you to be considered yours?

Do you consider yourself monogamous or polyamorous?

Why do you consider yourself monogamous/polyamorous?

How many submissives would you have, if you could have as many as you want?

**Why it's important:**

His answers may give you some indication of whether he is a Collector Dom, who is interested only in amassing a large number of subs or slaves without regard for anything else. It may also tell you something about his thinking in regards to collars, monogamy, polyamory, and the practicality of his ideas about living the lifestyle.

**How to interpret his answer:**

Evaluate his responses by placing them on a sliding scale between the following values, which should appear at each end of the spectrums, in this fashion:

Monogamous <----------------> Polyamorous

Practical <------------------------> Impractical

Experienced <-----------------> Inexperienced

Realistic <---------------------> Fantasy prone

Quality <-----------------------------> Quantity

**What you should do about it:**

It's rare that a complex issue like this one can be viewed as black and white. That's why evaluating his responses on a spectrum can be useful. Decide for yourself if what you see is compatible with what you seek in a partner.

**My Two Cents:**

Evelyn sat across the table from me at our local Starbucks, nursing a cappuccino and looking wistfully into my eyes as she asked dozens of questions about me, my writing, my life in general, and about my thoughts on the BDSM lifestyle. As much as I enjoyed gazing back into her beautiful blue eyes, I realized that it was time to interrupt our little reverie with a necessary dose of reality.

"I can see that you're interested in me," I said, chuckling. "So... this is probably a good time to tell you that I already have about ten girlfriends."

She blinked. "Ten? Seriously? You have *ten* girlfriends?"

I nodded. "More or less. Actually, it's probably closer to twelve, depending upon *your* definition of what constitutes a girlfriend." I waited for what typically happens next, which usually involves some variation of *bolting*.

She silently processed this information for a moment and then smiled mischievously. "Will you share? Can they be *my* girlfriends, too?"

I grinned and ordered us another round of coffee.

**Question #18:** Why are your former submissives no longer in a relationship with you?

**Follow-up questions:**

What were some of the things that drove you crazy about your former submissives?

What things about you drove *them* crazy?

Would any of them take you back if you were willing?

Was it your decision or theirs to end the relationship?

How did you release them?

Are you still friends with them?

**Why it's important:**

Here's where you learn a little more about what makes him tick and about what happens when the ticking *stops.*

**How to interpret his answer:**

Pay very close attention here. Anything that he says about his *former* submissives will also likely apply equally to his *future* submissives. Look for indications of megalomania, narcissism, delusion, or immaturity. How he talks about his exes may very well be how he talks about *you* someday.

Tactfully probe for specific information regarding his former partners and the relationship dynamic he had with them.

**What you should do about it:**

Look for similarities between his former partners and yourself. Take note of signs of selfishness or immaturity in his previous dynamics and assign yellow or red flags as appropriate.

**My Two Cents:**

Breaking up is hard to do. Getting that old Neal Sedaka song out of your head can be pretty damn hard to do, too.

Most people would probably guess, based solely on the many stories about my former submissives in this book, that I must *enjoy* talking about my exes. *I don't*.

I view each and every break-up as a personal failure on my part and frankly, I don't like to fail at *anything* that I do. Consequently, revisiting and retelling some of these stories can be discomforting, to say the least. It's not something that I'm typically willing to do unless there's a darn good reason for it. I just hope that it may help you to avoid some of the train wrecks that I was unable to.

It's also hard because I worry about how I portray some of my exes. There are only so many pages that can be devoted to each little story and there are always going to be parts that must be jettisoned for the sake of brevity. As a result, some people start looking like two-dimensional *caricatures* of their true selves. It's like seeing them through a carnival mirror that warps and distorts their appearance. That is a shame because they were each, in their own unique way, intelligent, engaging, complex, and amazing women. It just *kills* me that you'll never be able to know and appreciate them as I did. It really *isn't* fair, to them *or* to you.

On the other hand, it would be an even greater shame if the pain we endured turned out to be all for nothing. And so I tell these little stories and hope they help... *someone*.

**Question #19:** If I were to have a conversation about you with one of your former submissives, what would he or she tell me?

**Follow-up questions:**

Why do you think she would tell me that?

May I have a conversation about you with one of your former submissives?

Are the two of you still on good terms?

Why or why not?

**Why it's important:**

This is not an entirely hypothetical question. The BDSM culture is a small world, and sooner or later, you just might end up meeting one of his former submissives. This could turn out to be a goldmine of information, or a nightmare of epic proportions. Knowing how you should react when and if the opportunity arises is imperative.

**How to interpret his answer:**

Frankly, no one really knows what someone else would or wouldn't say about them privately, so any response that you get to that question will be pure conjecture. Even so, it is his conjecture that will tell you a lot about him, since it is typically human nature to project onto others what we may be subconsciously thinking about ourselves. Additionally, if he tells you that you may not ask his former subs about him, it may well be that he has something to hide.

**What you should do about it:**

If you *do* get permission to ask a former sub about him, decide for yourself whether it's going to be worth the hassle and emotional turmoil that will likely follow. He will probably see your request as a sign of your distrust, so tread lightly here.

**My Two Cents:**

"I just had a wonderful little chat with your former sub Lily," gushed Leilani. "Thank you for allowing me to have a chat with her. She is just delightful! I can see why you adored her so much!"

I smiled and said, "Yes, she's very sweet. I was really very sad to have to release her."

Leilani sat at my feet and laid her head upon my lap as I stroked her long black hair. After a moment of reflection, she asked, "Sir, would you mind telling me *why* you released her? You both still seem to be very fond of each other. What happened?"

I mulled my response a bit before replying, "It's true, I adored her then, and I still do. But I had to release her because she turned out to be an askhole."

Leilani raised her head and looked at me with a puzzled expression. "An... *askhole?* What in blue blazes is an askhole?"

"An askhole," I replied, "is someone who constantly asks you for your advice, but *never follows it.*"

**Question #20:** Do you know anyone who would be willing to provide references or vouch for you?

**Follow-up questions:**

How do these individuals know you?

What do you think they will tell me about you?

**Why it's important:**

Anyone who has been in the BDSM lifestyle for any significant length of time will have *some* kind of references, even if it is just a few friends. References help to establish his credibility.

**How to interpret his answer:**

A reluctance to provide any sort of references should be considered at least a yellow flag.

**What you should do about it:**

Ask for references and take any excuse for having no one who'll vouch for him with a huge grain of salt. Contact each of the references he provides, but make a reasonable effort to ensure that they are each legitimate, real individuals, and not just sock-puppet social media accounts controlled by the prospective Dominant, *himself*.

**My Two Cents:**

"How do I know that you're really who you say you are?" asked the woman I'd just "met" in a Facebook chat.

I pondered the question for a moment before replying, "I guess you don't. Is it important? I mean, it's not like I'm asking you out on a date, or anything."

She replied, "You could be someone pretending to be Michael Makai. I have a hard time believing that the real Mr. Makai would respond to a random chat request from a stranger, as *you* just did."

I replied, "I guess I could send you a photograph or something." I sent her a photo of myself that I'd taken earlier in the day while out hiking.

"Ha!" she scoffed, "Anyone could have gotten that picture off the internet! You'll have to do better than *that!*"

I was stumped. How do I prove that I am me, without divulging privileged information to complete strangers? The thought that I could ever be the victim of online impersonation had simply never occurred to me before. Why in the world would someone want to pretend to be me? And how do I prove that I really am me?

I finally resorted to Facebook. I asked some of my real-life friends on Facebook friends to vouch for me publicly. One of them said that I was the "real deal" and that he'd just had lunch with me. Another said, "The world couldn't handle more than one of you, Mike!" Still another said, "If I were going to impersonate someone, I'd impersonate someone *taller and better looking!*"

It's good to have friends who'll vouch for you, even if they're smart-asses.

**Question #22:** Would you still be interested in me, even if I told you there would be no sex?

**Follow-up questions:**

How important is sex to you in your relationships?

**Why it's important:**

Regardless of how important sex is to you personally, it can be extremely useful to know how important it is to your prospective Dominant.

**How to interpret his answer:**

Anyone who tells you that sex isn't important *at all* has about a 90% probability of being completely full of *crapola. Yes*, there *are* asexual people out there and some of them are *awesome people,* but unless that's what you're looking for in a relationship, this answer should be treated as a yellow flag.

**What you should do about it:**

Compare his answers with your personal beliefs about the importance of sex in a relationship. As you move forward, watch for actions, requests, and behaviors that seem to contradict what he has told you in response to this question.

**My Two Cents:**

My first real experience with a D/s relationship dynamic was relatively short-lived. It lasted about fifteen minutes.

I was an arrogant college student, working as a waiter in an upscale restaurant and dating one of my co-workers, an attractive 30-year old single mom whose *real name* was Sheree. Our relationship turned sexual rather quickly and that's where much of our energy seemed to be focused whenever we spent time together. That was just fine with me, but Sheree was beginning to want more out of the relationship.

One evening, after a long and frustrating work shift, we went to her apartment and collapsed onto her bed, seeking comfort in each other's arms. I started to unbutton her blouse, but she pushed my hand away and said, "That's all you're interested in, isn't it? It's all about the sex. You're not really interested in me, as a person. All you care about is getting laid."

What she said *angered* me. It angered me a *lot*. She'd been the one who made the first sexual advances in our relationship. She was the one who invited me into her bedroom practically every night after work. She was sexually insatiable, often desiring sex two or three times a day and wanting to try new and exciting things out in bed.

Yet *now*, here she was, telling me that it was all *I* cared about. That it was all just *me*. Frankly, that *pissed me off.*

Yes, I realize now, decades later, what she was really trying to say; what she was trying to do. Hindsight really *is* 20-20, even when you're looking through lenses coated with the dust of nearly four decades. She was trying to say that she wanted *more* than *just* sex from me.

She wanted a deeper relationship. But I was just nineteen years old and relatively inexperienced in relationships. I hadn't interpreted it that way at all. I thought she was trying to say that sex wasn't important to her, an assertion that I knew to be patently false. And so, like a complete *jerk*, I set out to prove her wrong.

I assured her that sex wasn't the only thing on my mind, and we moved on to other topics of discussion. Eventually, our cuddles turned into passion and, for the very first time in my life, I suggested tying a woman to the bed. To my surprise, she embraced the idea enthusiastically.

I stripped her naked and positioned her face-up and spread-eagle on the bed. I loosely secured her wrists and ankles to the four corner posts using belts, straps, clothesline, and other materials I found around the apartment. I removed my own clothing and began caressing, teasing, and arousing her in the ways she loved. Before long, she was entirely consumed by wanton lust and writhing in passion.

"Do you want me, baby? Do you want *this?*" I asked, kneeling near her face and looking into her eyes as I stroked myself. "How *badly* do you want it?"

"Oh yes," she moaned, barely able to get the words out as she panted and moaned, struggling helplessly against her restraints. "Please! *Please*, I want it so badly."

"Imagine that," I said. "Earlier, you told me that all I cared about was getting laid. That seems a little like the pot calling the kettle black, don't you think?"

I stepped away from the bed and began getting dressed. The sudden shift in mood and circumstance sent Sheree reeling and into shock. She was struggling hard to understand what was happening and what I was saying.

She stammered, "What...? What are you doing? Where are you *going?"*

I finished getting dressed and walked over to the head of the bed to release her right wrist from the cuff.

I replied, "I'm showing you just *how* unimportant sex is to me. *Goodnight,* Sheree." And with that, I walked out the front door.

## **Author's Sidebar**

I was nineteen years old. Cut me a little slack here, please. Yes, I was an *ass-hat;* a *complete jerk.* I know that, *now.*

I've never told this story before to anyone, mainly because it paints such an unflattering picture of who and what I was at the time. No one likes to revisit the ugliest parts of their past or to admit that they were stupid and wrong.

This is for Sheree: You probably don't even remember me, but I definitely remember *you.* On the astronomically improbable chance that you will ever read this, I just want to say that I am profoundly sorry for what I did to you that day, nearly forty years ago. For decades, I have wanted to apologize for my actions, but had no idea how to do it. I suppose this will have to *do.* Please forgive me.

And thank you, for introducing me to *bondage.*

**Question #23:** Tell me something about your religious or moral belief system.

**Follow-up questions:**

What religion are you? How long have you been a part of that religion?

How important is it that your partner shares your beliefs?

How tolerant of other religious beliefs are you?

What would you say if you knew that I was a (insert your religion here)?

How do you feel about discussing, defending, evangelizing, or arguing about religion?

**Why it's important:**

Religion is and always will be a dangerous minefield for relationships of any kind, whether they are D/s or vanilla. You may be open-minded, tolerant, or even supportive of other people's beliefs, but not everyone is. Some people truly believe that they are religiously tolerant until they run into something that they really disagree with. Others somehow think that "tolerating" your beliefs shouldn't necessarily prevent them from belittling or ridiculing them.

**How to interpret his answer:**

Compare not only his beliefs with your own for long-term compatibility, but examine closely his attitudes regarding religious tolerance or any lack thereof.

**What you should do about it:**

Decide for yourself whether you are tolerant of religious intolerance, or vice-versa.

**My Two Cents:**

Gloria was like a determined pit bull, unwilling to let go of something, once she'd sunk her teeth into it. "But why won't you tell me more about your religious beliefs, Sir?" she asked for the umpteenth time.

"As I've already told you," I replied, "I do *not* enjoy religious discussions or debates. No one is ever persuaded either way and it always ends up creating bad feelings all around. So, why bother starting down a path that leads us nowhere that we want to go?"

Gloria was undeterred. "But I don't want to debate with you; I just want to understand you better. I don't really have strong religious beliefs of my own, so it's not like I am going to argue with you. I care about you and I just enjoy learning all there is to know about you, whatever it happens to be!"

I was skeptical. Very skeptical. And what do I always do when I am skeptical of a statement? I find a way to test its veracity. And so I spent the next hour sharing my rather unique world-view and explaining what I considered to be the arcane secrets of life, the universe, god, and everything. And then I sat back and *waited* for it.

I didn't have to wait long.

"I thought you were smart," she said, her words dripping with sarcasm. "I don't know which is more disturbing, the fact that there are people out there who believe any of that, or that *you* do! How could anyone with even half a brain believe something so incredibly *stupid?"*

I laughed and said, "Are you referring to that bullshit you handed me earlier about how you would *never* ridicule the beliefs of others? I guess you're right, Gloria. I *was* stupid to believe you."

**Question #24:** Please tell me about your most recent real-life BDSM experience.

**Follow-up questions:**

When and where did it happen?

Was it a public scene?

Was it enjoyable to you?

Why or why wasn't it an enjoyable experience for you?

Is it something you'd want to do again?

How did your partner feel about it?

**Why it's important:**

This is one of those times where his claims of experience shouldn't be enough to satisfy you. You should ask for plenty of specifics, not only about what he has done, but about how things went. This is how you separate the wheat from the chaff or, in this case, the truth from the bullshit.

**How to interpret his answer:**

Any intentional vagueness or generalities in his response should be interpreted as an effort to deceive you.

**What you should do about it:**

Use your gut or intuition to determine whether he is being deliberately evasive in order to mask his inexperience. If you think so, consider that a yellow flag. Do keep in mind, however, the fact that many people in the lifestyle will be reluctant to share details of their BDSM experiences if it might expose sensitive information about themselves or others.

**My Two Cents:**

Peri was a young, attractive submissive who was relatively new to the lifestyle. She'd met a guy, and was interested in him as a prospective Dominant, but she couldn't shake the feeling that he was really just a vanilla guy who had developed an instant interest in the BDSM lifestyle upon learning that she considered herself a submissive.

Her gut feeling was that he was simply trying to bluff his way into her panties, but she just wasn't sure. So she brought him to meet me. She'd told him I was a sort of surrogate father-figure and that she was just excited about introducing him to me. The truth was she wanted me to vet the young man for her.

Our conversation was pleasant and informative. He seemed to be rather naive about the lifestyle, but there's no crime in that as long as you're not trying to pass as some sort of expert. As our conversation progressed, I began to notice an odd tendency for one-upsmanship. It didn't matter what anyone mentioned having ever done, he always had to mention that he'd done it better, harder, more often, or with greater expertise. Once I realized that he was treating the discussion as some sort of competition, I decided to test just how far he'd go to *win* it.

I told him the story of my former submissive who was an extreme masochist and my apparent misunderstanding, at the time, of what that really meant. The tale, which I wrote about in another book, involved a submissive who wanted me to pound nails through her nipples with a hammer and safety-pin her vagina closed. I explained that I'd learned about a hard limit that day that I never even knew I *had*.

Determined not to be outdone, the young man reached deep into his fertile imagination for something that would be able to top my story.

He suddenly and, apparently without much forethought, announced to us, "Hell, that wouldn't bother me! I'm a necrophiliac!"

At least the follow-up questions turned out to be extremely entertaining, if not particularly convincing.

**Question #25:** What are your thoughts on lifestyle protocols in general?

**Follow-up questions:**

How familiar are you with common lifestyle protocols?

How important are they to you?

Why do you feel the way you do about them?

**Why it's important:**

Protocols, which are simply customs, courtesies, and good manners for people who subscribe to the lifestyle, are a big deal in the fetish culture. Even if you couldn't care less about protocols in general, there are always going to be enough people in the BDSM lifestyle who do that it could conceivably become a problem that affects both of you in the future, especially if you're perceived by others as a couple.

**How to interpret his answer:**

There really are only about three possible responses to this question. (1) I am old-school and believe strongly in following protocols. (2) I'm ambivalent about them in general. Perhaps there is a time and place for them. (3) *Fuck* protocols! I make my *own* rules, and anyone who doesn't like that can kiss my ass!

**What you should do about it:**

Consider option three to be a yellow or perhaps even a red flag, depending upon your own personal viewpoint on this subject. It is not at all unusual for an individual to become a pariah and be banned from a local BDSM munch group for failure to follow basic protocols. If you are connected to that individual, something like that can have significant consequences for you, too.

**My Two Cents:**

I've seen it happen time and time again. The most recent time was just a few months ago, when a married couple named Tom and Marianne contacted me to ask why they were both suddenly being left off the invitation lists for various local munch group events.

I replied, "Why ask me, Tom? I'm not a member of the group's managing committee. You'd probably be better off asking someone who could give you an answer in some official capacity."

Tom, who seemed pretty exasperated by my question, said, "I would, if anyone would even talk to me. I can't seem to get a straight answer out of anyone. You're the only one who is returning my calls, and I trust your advice. Will *you* tell me what is going on?"

I sighed and told him the answer that no one else seemed willing to give him. "Your wife has violated the group's rules and protocols and then, when she was asked to stop doing that, she mounted a very nasty and public crusade against the committee members who dared to correct her. Tom, *you've* done nothing wrong and you are still welcome at all the events, but I guess the committee has just decided it would just be rude to invite you if your wife wasn't welcome to attend with you. I'm really sorry about that."

Tom looked down at his shoes and shook his head. "I was unaware of any of this," he said.

I shrugged and told him, "I wish I had a better answer for you, Tom. We do miss you at the events."

Tom turned to go home to his wife and as he did, I heard him growl under his breath, "*Somebody* is about to get a very painful lesson in protocol.*"*

**Question #26:** Do you consider yourself a Gorean?

**Follow-up questions:**

What do you know about the Gorean lifestyle?

If you are a Gorean, how seriously do you take the Gorean lifestyle?

Have you read any of the Gor novels by John Norman?

If so, what did you think of them?

**Why it's important:**

Perhaps you know nothing about Gor. Or maybe you *do*, but have an intense dislike for it. There are plenty of people in the lifestyle who cringe at the very mention of this D/s subculture. Maybe you just don't care much about it, at all.

Regardless, this question is important because Goreans share a world-view and philosophy that differs significantly from that of the mainstream BDSM culture. In fact, most Goreans do not consider themselves a part of the BDSM lifestyle at *all* and typically prefer to categorize themselves as being in a category all their own.

**How to interpret his answer:**

Before asking this question, spend some time familiarizing yourself with the Gorean subculture. Reading my previous work would be one way to do it. Another possible way is to search the internet for articles on Gorean traditions, training, and philosophy.

**What you should do about it:**

Once you've familiarized yourself with what is means to be a Gorean, ask him the question. Then, you'll be able to decide for yourself whether it resonates with you or gives you the *heebie-jeebies*.

**My Two Cents:**

I have a difficult time relating in any meaningful way to those who follow the Gorean way. Perhaps it's their intense adoration of the completely fictional culture of a planet that exists only in their imaginations and in the pages of John Norman's pulp fiction novels. Maybe it's their dogged memorization of the fictional animals, places, customs, fashions, and even the imaginary *language* of Gor. It's possible that it's simply the endless rabid arguments they have to earn bragging rights to being seen as the geekiest Goreans on *this* planet.

I'm a Star Wars fan, but I've never *once* had the urge to learn how to speak Wookie or to go around quizzing other people on how well *they* speak it. I love Dr. Who, but I don't keep a phony sonic screwdriver in my pocket or paint my house to resemble a tardis.

All things considered, I guess I'd make a lousy Gorean. I have a hard enough time making sense of *Earth* culture.

**Question #27:** Please tell me something about yourself that would probably surprise me.

**Follow-up questions:**

Why do you think that would surprise me?

Do you think you are misunderstood by most people?

**Why it's important:**

This question can be important for two reasons. First, you may be able to learn something about your prospective Dominant that you would never learn any other way, simply because you would never have thought to ask.

This question also gives you a glimpse of the phenomenon of social perception feedback loops. In other words, does his understanding of what people think about him bear any resemblance at all to what they *really* think about him?

You may think this is relatively unimportant until you hear him say something like, "Everyone hates me," or "Even my mother thinks I'm a psychopath!"

**How to interpret his answer:**

Enjoy learning something about him that you might not otherwise have discovered. The important thing here is you may get a peek at what he *thinks* is going on inside of *your* head or in the heads of the other people around him.

**What you should do about it:**

Allow him to believe that this question is more about your insatiable curiosity and learning something surprising about him, rather than a matter of mucking around in his social perceptual feedback loop.

## My Two Cents:

Occasionally, I vent my frustrations publicly in social media and today was one of those days. I was lamenting the fact that, when it came to debating important BDSM lifestyle issues in public forums, it seemed that it was always the least knowledgeable individuals who had the *most* to say on any given subject.

In response to my public rant, my friend Chris in Houston sent me a message saying, "You are describing something called the *Dunning-Kruger Effect*. Look it up, my friend!" And so I did.

I was amazed that this phenomenon not only had a name, but it had been scientifically tested and proven again and again. The initial study was inspired by a man named McArthur Wheeler, who robbed two banks after covering his face with lemon juice, because he actually thought it would prevent his face from being recorded on the bank's surveillance cameras.

The scientific study (and several other studies which followed) showed that it was always the *least* competent people who consistently rated their competency the *highest*. When test subjects were given tests to complete and then asked to guess their scores, the ones with an average score in the 12th percentile consistently estimated themselves to be at the 62nd percentile.

Conversely, the individuals with real knowledge, who scored very *well* on the tests, consistently *underestimated* their own competence. They erroneously assumed that just because the test was easy for them, it must also have been easy for everyone else!

Charles Darwin summed it up rather nicely when he wrote, "Ignorance more frequently begets confidence than does knowledge."

**Question #28:** Are you a clingy, jealous, or suspicious Dominant?

**Follow-up questions:**

Are you very possessive? Why or why not?

What are the kinds of things that typically upset you?

Have you been betrayed by a partner in the past?

If so, how did that make you feel?

What sorts of things cause you to become suspicious?

**Why it's important:**

Depending on your outlook on life and relationships, this is the sort of issue that can make or break your dynamic.

**How to interpret his answer:**

Don't expect to get a response to this question that is entirely accurate or truthful. It's not at all unusual for some people to be largely unaware of just *how* clingy, jealous, or suspicious they can be.

**What you should do about it:**

Evaluate anything he says about not having any of those qualities with a large dose of skepticism. Observe his behavior going forward to see if it is consistent with his own self-evaluation in this regard.

**My Two Cents:**

"Master," asked Kitten, "Don't you *ever* get jealous?"

I shrugged and replied, "Everyone gets jealous, babe."

She furrowed her brow and said, "But I've never seen you get jealous, Master! Not even when you have good reason to be. Why *is* that?"

I pondered the question a bit before answering, "Jealousy is just a feeling. It's usually all about the good time you think someone else is having, or being afraid of *losing* something or someone. It's human nature and perfectly normal to feel a certain amount of jealousy, but what's important is what you do about it."

"So, what do *you* do about it when *you* feel jealous?" she asked.

"I suppose it depends entirely on the situation," I replied. "Whatever it is I decide to do, I try to ensure that it isn't going to be counter-productive or damaging to my relationship dynamic. Sometimes, our insecurities or jealousy can end up being the very cause of whatever it is we most afraid of happening. In essence, it becomes a *self-fulfilling prophecy.*"

"So," she teased, "Does that mean I can go out to dinner with Matthew, that guy I met the other day?"

"Sure." I replied, "As long as he buys me dinner, *too.*"

**Question #29:** Have you ever been a switch or a submissive?

**Follow-up questions:**

If so, why did you change your D/s orientation?

Have you ever considered becoming a switch or submissive?

How would you feel if *I* was a switch?

Have you ever been involved with a switch in the past?

If so, how did that go?

**Why it's important:**

Your prospective Dominant may still be finding his way when it comes to his true role in the BDSM lifestyle. Some people subscribe to the belief that you can't be a good Dom unless you've been a good submissive first. Others believe that if you've ever been a submissive, you'll never truly be a good Dominant.

It is also very common even for experienced members of the BDSM lifestyle to confuse being a Dominant with being a Top, or to confuse being a submissive with being a bottom.

**How to interpret his answer:**

If you are one of the people who is confused about the difference between being a Dominant and Topping, or the difference between being a submissive and bottoming, do a little homework before tackling this question.

The glossary at the end of this book can give you a cursory explanation. For a more detailed treatment of this subject, refer to my previous works.

**What you should do about it:**

Once you've done your homework, evaluate his responses to this set of questions through the prism of your beliefs regarding what qualifies someone as a true Dominant, and about whether Doms are made or born.

There are some submissives who cannot stand even the merest hint of submission in their Dominants. Others are able to embrace the submissive side of their Doms as a sign that he understands her feelings and where she may be coming from.

Give some serious thought to how you feel about it and what you believe, educate him as necessary so you can discuss this issue in a meaningful way, and then decide whether his responses match your expectations and needs.

**My Two Cents:**

"I need some advice," said my friend Roxanne, as she took a seat at my table in the coffee shop.

"Advice about what, exactly?" I asked.

She replied, "There's this Dominant who's been using Facebook to communicate daily with me. I've haven't met him yet, even though he says he is local. He says he wants a chance to meet me and to show me that he would make a good Master for me."

"Okay," I said. "So, what's the problem?"

"He must have a terrible memory," she said, shaking her head. "He obviously doesn't remember *me*, but I remember *him* from several months ago, when he was messaging me, calling me Mistress and begging me practically every day for a chance to lick my boots!"

"Okay," I said, once again. "So, what's the problem?"

She seemed a little perplexed. "Well, what the hell am I supposed to do about it?"

"That depends," I replied. "How do you feel about it?"

She deliberated for a moment before responding, "I could *never, ever* submit to man who, just five months ago, was begging me for a chance to lick my boots. Not in a million fucking years."

"Okay," I said, nodding. "So, what's the problem?"

"Ugh!" she said, rolling her eyes and throwing up her hands in utter frustration. "Talking to you is like being stuck on some swamp planet with BDSM Yoda!"

"Learning *quickly*, you are," I replied, ever so sagely.

**Question #30:** Who knows that you are a Dominant in this lifestyle?

**Follow-up questions:**

Do your friends know?

Does your family know?

Do any of your coworkers and associates know?

What steps, if any, do you take to protect your privacy?

**Why it's important:**

Knowing this information can help you to assist him in protecting his privacy. It will also give you a better idea how much of his kink life is integrated into his day to day personal life.

**How to interpret his answer:**

Take his response at face-value. It's difficult to imagine why anyone might want to fudge the facts on this subject.

**What you should do about it:**

Resolve to respect and protect his privacy as appropriate. You should never "out" someone without his or her consent. Not only would doing so violate a very sacred principle of the lifestyle, but you should never forget that it can be a double-edged sword that cuts both ways.

Never assume that you can wreak havoc in someone's life and that they will do nothing in retaliation. This is doubly true if you've already ascertained that the person is a jerk. He just may turn out to be a very resourceful jerk who can not only find you very easily, no matter how anonymous you think you are, but just might burn your house down.

It *happens*. Don't ever think it couldn't happen to you.

**My Two Cents:**

I told this story in a previous work, but at the risk of sounding like a broken record, I think it bears repeating, again and again, until people understand that they are not *ever* truly anonymous.

"How's your trial with your new Master going?" I asked my young friend Roxy. She'd met Drago in this very chatroom just a week earlier and had agreed to a collar of consideration from him after just a few minutes of conversation. At the time, I'd considered it an extremely unwise decision, but it wasn't my place to say so.

Roxy was silent for a moment and then replied, "Not well. In fact, I told him to *go fuck himself*."

Not entirely unexpected, I thought. She was a young and inexperienced brat. He was a hard-core Gorean. Typically not a very good combination. "I'm sorry to hear that, hon. I'm guessing the trial is off, then?"

She gave a little nod and replied, "I guess so. He threatened me. Do you think I should be worried?"

If *she* wasn't, I was. "What do you mean, threatened you?" I asked. "What did he say, *exactly?*"

Roxy replied, "He said he would hunt me down in real-life and make me sorry that I had spoken to him like that." Long pause. "He can't really *do* that, can he?"

"I'm pretty sure he could accomplish it, if he really wanted to." I said.

Clearly, she didn't like what she was hearing. "Are you saying that he really could find out where I live? There is no possible way! I have never even told him what state I live in. At most, he knows my first name, and that isn't even my real first name, it's just a nickname."

I sighed. I have always hated the painful process convincing someone that she isn't really as clever or as anonymous as she thinks she is. "Don't go anywhere," I said. "I'll be back in five minutes."

When I returned, I showed her what I'd found: Her full legal name. Her home address, landline *and* cell phone numbers. I'd found her email address, Facebook, Pinterest *and* Tumblr accounts.

I showed Roxy pictures of her recent Jamaican vacation and gave her the names of all her family members, pets, and best friends. And I'd found it *all* in less than five minutes.

Suddenly, Roxy wasn't feeling quite so invincible.

**Question #31:** If I were willing to meet you, would you want to meet me in real life?

**Follow-up questions:**

If not, why not?

If not, where do you expect this relationship to go from here?

If so, how soon would you want to meet me?

If so, where would you want to meet, and under what circumstances?

If so, would you be expecting our meeting to involve sex?

How would you feel about meeting if there was going to be no sex involved?

How would you feel about meeting if I brought a friend along with me?

Have you ever met someone in real-life after getting to know them online before?

How did that go?

**Why it's important:**

First meetings are difficult and stressful even under the best of circumstances. If you do, indeed, have an interest in meeting your prospective Dominant face to face, knowing his thoughts on this issue will be paramount.

**How to interpret his answer:**

Pay very close attention to his response, and make every attempt to read between the lines as necessary. It is common for people, both Doms and subs, to have completely unrealistic notions of what a first meeting will be like, and there will almost always be unspoken misconceptions or expectations.

Sometimes, these mistaken expectations are simply awkward or disappointing. Other times, they can turn into an ugly or even potentially dangerous situation.

Be sure to avoid allowing him to misinterpret the question as an *invitation* to meet you face-to-face. Reemphasize the hypothetical nature of the question, if necessary.

**What you should do about it:**

Explore this issue with your prospective Dom at great length. Do *not* drop the subject until you are completely satisfied that you are both on the same sheet of music regarding both of your expectations for a first meeting. For a more complete, in-depth discussion of this topic, I highly recommend you read the "First Meetings" chapter of my book, "Domination & Submission: The BDSM Relationship Handbook."

**My Two Cents:**

Eve, my submissive, was excited about having made a new local Facebook friend named Roger, and had agreed to meet him for the first time for dinner. Now, I'm not a particularly jealous Master, and I typically don't try to tell my submissives who their friends should be. I also realize that sometimes dinner is just dinner, and nothing more. Even so, I do try to look out for the safety of my girls to the best of my ability. This day was no exception.

"That's nice, babe!" I replied. "Where are you going to dinner? Is he picking you up or are you meeting him somewhere?"

She wrinkled her brow in thought and said, "Hmmm. Let me check." She pulled out her phone and recited the address to which she would be going later that evening. "He told me to meet him at 2010 Cherry Avenue, on the west side of town."

I nodded and pulled out my phone. Google Earth is my friend. A few taps on the screen, and I was looking at a street-view of Roger's modest home.

Suddenly, my skepticism was showing. "Are you seriously telling me that this guy expects you to go straight to his house for your first face to face meeting?"

She frowned. *"Rut roh...* Kinda looks like it, doesn't it?"

I nodded and said, "So, here's what you're going to do. You're going to text Roger right now and you're going to explain that your dinner date for tonight has been summarily cancelled by your Master because he didn't have the good sense to arrange to meet you safely in a public place. Go ahead and tell him that now, word for word. If he is going to be your friend, even a completely vanilla friend, he is going to have to get used to the fact that you have a Master who not only takes your safety very seriously, but will hold him personally accountable for it."

She texted the message to him and, to his credit, he seemed to take it in stride. Eve, on the other hand, was chagrined and horrified about having almost made a potentially dangerous mistake. I told her that she should just chalk it up to experience and that as long as she learned something from the experience, then it was a good thing.

I figured I'd tell her *later* about coming along as her chaperone for their *next* date.

**Question #32:** What are your thoughts on a submissive's hard and soft limits?

**Follow-up questions:**

Do you use a safe word?

Has a bottom ever had to safe-word out of a scene with you?

Please tell me about the last time that a safe-word was used by a bottom under your control in a scene.

**Why it's important:**

Everyone has limits, whether they like to admit it or not. Failure to respect a person's limits is almost always going to be a very serious problem. Consent, in this lifestyle, is everything. Violating a person's limits is a violation of his or her consent, especially if those limits have been previously discussed and understood. Obviously, violating a limit that you are unaware of becomes just a bit more problematic, since no one should be expected to be a mind reader. Even so, you should never lose sight of the fact that any failure to respect limits is a betrayal of trust, and that practically any sexual act performed without your partner's consent can and often will be considered a case of sexual assault or rape.

**How to interpret his answer:**

Anyone who says that he doesn't believe in limits or doesn't use safe words is a potentially dangerous person. Some couples who engage in BDSM play as a couple frequently or exclusively can become very adept at reading each other's verbal and nonverbal communication. In those cases, a rational case can be made for not using a formal safeword mainly because they are simply employing a less formal method of accomplishing exactly the same thing. Similarly, once a couple establishes a stable and trusting real-world relationship, it is often the case that some limits have a funny way of just fading away.

None of this should serve to justify a prospective Dominant who attempts to tell you that safe words are unnecessary, or that your limits should not be respected just because he considers it his solemn duty to "push your limits."

**What you should do about it:**

Run, don't walk, away from anyone who does not respect the notion of hard and soft limits or claims that it is his duty to push your limits in any way that violates your consent. Be very wary of anyone who doesn't use safe words, but understand that some long-time couples who know each other well may not have much of a need for them. Even so, if you're at a point where you are still just interviewing a prospective Dominant that probably doesn't apply to you.

**My Two Cents:**

Cathy and I had been in a D/s relationship for several months, and BDSM play had always been an integral part of our relationship. We typically relied upon the simple and familiar "red, yellow, green" system that many people in the BDSM lifestyle employ.

Red means there needs to be an immediate halt to all activity now, unconditionally and with no need for explanations or excuses. Yellow means slow down or reduce the intensity of whatever it is you're doing. Green means "keep up the good work!"

One afternoon, we decided to experiment a bit with some predicament bondage. Predicament bondage is basically a matter of placing someone into restraints in such a way that there is no possible way to get comfortable. It isn't always painful, but it is, almost by definition, always going to be uncomfortable.

On this particular day, I decided to restrain Cathy in such a way that she was standing naked, facing me with her ankles attached to a spreader bar, her back severely arched, her arms in cuffs above her, and blindfolded with her face turned up towards the ceiling.

In retrospect, all I can say is it seemed like a good idea at the time.

There was no doubt in my mind that this position was going to be profoundly uncomfortable for Cathy. That was, after all, the whole idea. I also knew that she wasn't going to experience any significant pain, and that she wouldn't be injured in any way. Nevertheless, I kept a close eye on her as I applied some light flogging and cropping to her sensitive areas, which she seemed to enjoy immensely.

After a few minutes of this, I noticed that something wasn't quite right and immediately informed her that I needed discontinue the flogging and release her from her restraints. She was very disappointed, but followed my instructions as I unbuckled her wrist and ankle cuffs, quickly removed her blindfold, and directed her to sit down as I placed a light blanket around her shoulders.

"Master, why did we have to stop?" she asked, plaintively. "I was really enjoying that!"

I replied, "We needed to stop because you weren't looking well. The position I put you in must've triggered some sort of adverse physiological reaction."

"That's weird, Master." she said, frowning. "I can't imagine why you thought I wasn't doing okay, because I feel just fi..."

Suddenly, in mid-sentence, she stopped, grimaced, and made an odd sound that was a cross between a burp and a growl. Then she looked at me, her eyes wide with surprise, and said, "Oh no! I think I'm going to *throw up!*"

Later, after her nausea passed and she was resting safely in bed, she propped herself up on one elbow and asked, "Master, how did you know that I was going to be sick even before I knew?"

I laughed and told her, "Baby, I'm pretty used to seeing your pulse and respiration go from one extreme to another while we play. I've grown accustomed to seeing you squirm, quiver, shake, rattle, and roll. But today was the first time that I have ever seen you turn fifty shades of *green!*"

**Question #33:** What are *your* hard and soft limits?

**Follow-up questions:**

Do you have any BDSM or role-play limits?

Do you have any sexual limits?

**Why it's important:**

Surprise! Even Dominants have limits. While this may not be an issue that comes up terribly often, it *is* common enough that it definitely should be discussed. It's entirely possible that your prospective Dominant has limits that he isn't even aware of, simply because it's a subject that's never come up in the past. Learning what they are now will save you both the pain and embarrassment of learning about them after it's too late.

**How to interpret his answer:**

If your prospective dominant attempts to claim that he has no limits, you should ask a few probing questions to test that hypothesis.

Would it be acceptable for you to don a strap-on dildo and peg him anally? Are you allowed to cut him with a knife, hold a loaded gun to his head, or choke him until he passes out? Are you allowed to invite other males to participate in a sexual threesome with the two of you? Would he be willing to drive nails through your nipples with a hammer or safety-pin your vagina closed? What if you wanted to stick a urethral probe into his penis or engage in some other form of cock & ball torture? Chances are pretty good that at least one of these questions will elicit a response consisting of "Not just no, but *hell no!"* And that's how you disprove the urban myth of the so-called no-limits Dom.

**What you should do about it:**

If he continues to insist that he has no limits whatsoever, there can be only two real possibilities, neither of which makes him a very good candidate. The first possibility is that he is lying, deluded, or both. The second is that he is a psychopath.

On the other hand, if you *do* end up having a frank discussion about his hard and soft limits, consider it a healthy development and a rare peek into his head you might not have gotten any other way.

**My Two Cents:**

My good friend Jessica just *loves* having this discussion with prospective Dominants who attempt to portray themselves as hard-core BDSM lifestylers by claiming to have *no limits*. Her response is almost always some variation of the following:

"So, what you're *saying* is, I can grind your balls under my stiletto heel and you won't mind at all? Because if that's *so*, I think we should get started *right now*. I've had a really bad day, and I'm seriously ready to take it out on some *dumb motherfucker* who thinks he's too *macho* to have any limits!"

Needless to say, most don't stick around long enough for her to go get her stilettos.

**Question #34:** What kind of Dominant are you?

**Follow-up questions:**

What is it you enjoy most about your role as a Dominant?

Are you kind or harsh?

Are you a sadist? How much of a sadist?

Are you a masochist? How much of a masochist?

**Why it's important:**

There are many different kinds of Dominants. One size doesn't fit all. If you are a masochist, for example, you might do well to seek out a Sadistic Dom. A Kajira might want to find a Gorean Master. Each submissive type has one or two ideal corresponding Dominant types. A mismatch is no guarantee of failure, but it can definitely make life far more difficult than it needs to be.

**How to interpret his answer:**

If you are unfamiliar with the most common categories of Dominants and submissives, I highly recommend that you refer to the first chapters of "Domination & Submission."

At the very least, listen carefully to his rationale for categorizing himself as he does. Be prepared to probe well beyond the same old tired clichés that phony Dominants use but are meaningless. They include all-time favorites like: "I am strict, but fair" or "I am a loving Dominant."

**What you should do about it:**

Know first who and what *you* are, before embarking on a quest to find the perfect Dominant for you. Educate yourself, and if necessary, educate your prospective Dominant before diving head-first into this discussion.

If, after having this talk, it becomes readily apparent that the two of you are going to be a mismatch, consider cutting your losses and moving on *now*, rather than putting yourselves through months or even years of potential grief.

**My Two Cents:**

"He seems to take constant delight in being unnecessarily *mean* to me," Layla grouched, poking at her food. "It hurts my feelings and makes me feel like shit. Can't you *talk* to him? He respects you. Couldn't you just explain to him that Littles like me need lots of love and cuddles?"

"Layla," I replied, "He's a sadist."

"I know that, Sir," she said. "But *why* does he always have to be so *cruel* to me?"

This time around, I said it with more emphasis. *"Because he's a sadist.* Layla, that's what sadists *do*. The very definition of a sadist is someone who takes pleasure in being cruel or inflicting pain on others. You knew he was a sadist going in. You bragged about it, for crying out loud! You are not going to be able change that about him. You really only have two choices: you can accept him for what he is or you can walk away."

Three months later, she chose to walk away.

**Question #35:** Have you ever seriously hurt someone?

**Follow-up questions:**

If so, was it intentional or unintentional?

Have you ever fantasized about seriously hurting someone?

Do you feel you are capable of seriously hurting someone?

Why or why not?

**Why it's important:**

It's important because it *sucks* to get hurt. A Dominant who misjudges his own skill level or ability is likely to hurt someone. You don't want to wait until you're in the back of an ambulance and on your way to the emergency room to learn that your prospective Dominant is clueless, or even worse, a psychopath who fantasizes about seriously injuring, maiming, or even killing another human being for his own twisted pleasure.

**How to interpret his answer:**

If he says he fantasizes about seriously hurting someone, believe it. This is not something any rational person *jokes* about.

**What you should do about it:**

Treat any incident involving injuries as a yellow flag. Treat any pattern of injuries as a red flag. Consider anyone who fantasizes about causing serious bodily harm to other human beings as a potentially dangerous individual.

**My Two Cents:**

It's sometimes difficult to imagine that there really are people out there who not only fantasize about maiming or even killing their fellow human beings, but sometimes actually *do* those kinds of things.

When I was a young soldier in the army, I was stationed at Baumholder, West Germany for ten long years. For part of that time, I was attached to the 2nd Battalion, 68th Armor Regiment, where I was told some crazy stories about a guy who'd transferred out of the unit shortly before I arrived.

Jeff had been assigned to my battalion as an army medic. It was rumored that he'd been accused of drugging and raping a fellow male soldier, but there hadn't been enough evidence to convict him, so the charges were dropped. The army wanted him gone, and eventually they discharged him for alcohol abuse. The story made for good barracks scuttlebutt, but it wasn't until several years later that I finally made the connection between the young man that I'd heard so much about and the newspaper headlines.

Jeff, the army medic in my battalion, was a murderer, necrophiliac, and cannibal responsible for the deaths of at *least* seventeen people.

When he was arrested in Wisconsin, police found four severed heads in his kitchen, seven human skulls in his bedroom, and two human hearts in his refrigerator. Elsewhere in his apartment, they found two skeletons, a pair of severed hands, two severed penises, and three dismembered torsos.

He was obsessed with drugging his victims and then drilling holes into their skulls so he could inject chemicals directly into their brains in an effort to produce compliant *sex slaves*.

The former Army medic's full name was Jeffrey Dahmer.

**Question #36:** What if it turned out that I was younger than I told you I was?

**Follow-up questions:**

How young would be too young?

What if it turned out that I was older than I told you I was?

How old would be too old?

**Why it's important:**

It *might* be important if you were lying about your age, but you'd never do *that*, would you? The real reason for asking this question is to reveal your prospective Dom's thinking, biases, and preferences as they pertain to *age*.

**How to interpret his answer:**

Listen carefully to how he reacts to the notion of someone fudging their age. This will tell you a lot about how scrupulously honest you will have to be with this person going forward.

Pay close attention to his response to the "how old is too old" portion of the question. Some men are so obsessed with youth and beauty that they'll discard their partners once they reach a certain age. His answer will not only tell you if he is one of those men, but it may even tell you his age limit.

On the other hand, if he doesn't have an answer to "how young is too young," he just might have pedophilic tendencies that you should be aware of.

**What you should do about it:**

Remember, he'll think this question is about lying. Let him continue to think so. If his responses lead you to think he may be an age-bigot or pedophile, consider it a red flag and move on to the next candidate.

**My Two Cents:**

I answered the Skype video call and there, on my laptop screen, was someone I'd never seen before.

Yes, I knew her; her voice was the same, but the face didn't match the many photos that Valerie had sent to me over the past few months. She was *clearly* not the 25 year-old that she'd described herself as.

She was sobbing. Her face was swollen and red. "I am so, so sorry, Sir." she sobbed. "This is the real me. I'm not 25 years old, I'm 47 years old. The sexy lingerie pictures I sent to you were pictures of my *daughter*, not me. She gave me those pictures because I told her I wanted to play a joke on someone. Everything else that I told you about myself was true. I'm still the same person!"

"No, Valerie," I said, "You're not. Not even close. What did you hope to accomplish? Where in the world did you think this was all going to end up?"

"I... I... don't know!" she cried. "Please, Sir! Please give me another chance! I love you! I never meant to hurt you! Please give me a chance to prove to you that I'm still the same person. I'm *begging* you, Sir!"

I shook my head and replied, "Frankly, I don't know how I could ever trust you again. We can never go back to what we thought we had. You impersonated your own daughter for three months, for crying out loud! I'm sorry, Valerie, but that's just *nuts*."

The video call, like the relationship, was now over.

**Question #37:** What BDSM Topping skills do you have?

**Follow-up questions:**

How did you learn them?

How proficient are you at them?

When was the last time you practiced those particular skills?

Was this done at a public BDSM play party?

What is it that you enjoy most about that activity?

Do you feel that it is important to have a submissive who is trained in bottoming skills?

What are your thoughts on providing aftercare following a BDSM scene?

**Why it's important:**

This question is important as a way to learn a little more about his preferences, topping abilities, experience levels, and BDSM philosophy in general.

**How to interpret his answer:**

Accept what he tells you at face value unless it reeks of obvious deception.

**What you should do about it:**

This is a great opportunity to learn something about his topping technique without necessarily having to experience it first-hand. Use this subject to start a conversation about your own bottoming skills and other proficiencies or to brainstorm a possible future BDSM scene that you'd like to try with him some day.

Consider any refusal to consider aftercare a necessary follow-up to a BDSM scene as a potential red flag.

## My Two Cents:

This particular topic happens to be a very serious pet peeve of mine. Part of the reason is my natural resentment of the notion that anyone can pick up a flogger, paddle, or a length of rope and pretend to be a Top. Part of the reason is I have seen first-hand exactly how incredibly *dangerous* that notion can be.

Many years ago, about five minutes after a particularly intense BDSM session with one of my partners, I noticed that she had some difficulty grasping an object with her left hand. I watched her more intently and saw that she seemed happy, but only half her mouth seemed to be smiling. I immediately rushed her to the hospital emergency room where we learned that, as a result of undiagnosed high blood pressure, she had suffered a hemorrhagic stroke.

It is unusual for a 36-year old woman to suffer a stroke, but it *happens*. Subsequent MRI scans showed a walnut-sized hemorrhage in the right side of her brain. The doctors told us that if she hadn't gotten to the emergency room on time, she could have died or ended up paralyzed for life. This was, as you might imagine, a serious wake-up call for us.

Fast forward twenty years to a BDSM play party held at the home of some local friends. Our wonderful hosts had a nicely equipped dungeon in their two-car garage, a dining room table piled high with brownies and other yummy snacks, and a roaring fire going in a backyard fire pit. There were perhaps fifteen people in attendance.

Late in the evening, a couple of my friends took center stage to do a scene. Dawg, a novice male Dominant, prepared to do a public flogging scene with Janie, an attractive Asian woman and a moderately experienced switch. By this time, several people had already moved out back to sit around the fire pit and chat.

The few of us who were still in the dungeon area watched the unfolding scene with some bemusement. Dawg had apparently never used a flogger before. Half the time, the flogger's falls didn't even make contact. The other half of the time, they struck Janie's body in the wrong areas or with inappropriate force.

Her growing frustration was fairly obvious to just about everyone in the room *except* Dawg. It was an agonizing and painful thing for any experienced Top to have to watch. Consequently, the few people who had been in the dungeon as spectators quietly slipped outside to join the growing group around the backyard fire pit. I was one of them. Twenty minutes later, Dawg joined us out there too.

I was immediately concerned and asked him, "Where's Janie?"

"Oh, she's still inside." he replied.

"You're not staying with her as part of her aftercare?" I asked. "She's not all alone in the house, is she?"

He shrugged. "Yeah, she's alone. But she said she didn't need any aftercare. She doesn't mind being alone. Besides, I needed a smoke."

To say that I was incensed would have been an extreme understatement. I leaned in close to him, my nose practically touching his, and told him, "You need to get your ass back in there *right now* and make sure that she is okay. Whether she *thinks* she needs aftercare or not is completely irrelevant. Your responsibility as her Top is to *be there*, keep an eye on her to ensure her well-being, and provide aftercare as needed. *You got that, Dawg?"*

He nodded silently, snuffed out his cigarette, and went back inside to check on Janie.

**Question #38:** Please tell me about some of your sexual fantasies.

**Follow-up questions:**

Do you think you'll ever want to try that in real-life?

What has stopped you from trying that in the past?

How have your previous partners felt about that particular fantasy?

Are there any sexual fantasies that you would be afraid to tell anyone about?

Are there any sexual fantasies that you would be afraid to try for any reason?

Would you be interested in learning about some of my sexual fantasies?

**Why it's important:**

Even though you can have BDSM without sex, and (obviously, for millions of vanilla folk) vice versa, most of us tend to like heaping helpings of both in the bedroom. This question can open windows of understanding to what motivates and arouses your prospective Dominant and spur future conversations that will enhance your relationship.

**How to interpret his answer:**

This is your golden opportunity to see just how much of this BDSM thing is just in his head. It's also a good way to assess his integration of sex and BDSM.

**What you should do about it:**

If he says that he has fantasies that he is afraid to tell anyone about you should consider that a possible yellow flag, but don't badger him for details. Consider it a win that he has told you *that* much.

If he tells you that he would like to learn more about your sexual fantasies, take the opportunity to throw him a bone, but do not get caught up in making this all about yourself by spilling your guts in a tell-all fantasy extravaganza. Keep your eye on the ball and try to stay focused on learning what you can about him.

**My Two Cents:**

Jenna had been quizzing me all evening and got around to asking me, "What are your sexual fantasies?"

"I really don't have any," I replied, and waited for what inevitably comes next. After all, it isn't as if I haven't already *had* this conversation over a hundred times.

"Huh?" she said. "How can you not have any sexual fantasies? I call *bullshit*."

"It is what it is," I said. "I've been lucky enough to have opportunities to fulfill all my fantasies. I once took one of those silly tests listing your sexual experiences and the only one I'd never tried before was *armpit sex.*"

The look of incredulity on her face caused me to shrug sheepishly, adding, "There *is* such a thing. Who *knew?*"

**Question #39:** What's wrong with you?

**Follow-up questions:**

What would you consider to be your greatest flaws or weaknesses?

What, if anything, do you think has stopped you from being as successful as you want in life thus far?

Do you suffer from any mental illnesses?

Do you have any anger issues?

If so, what makes you angry and how do you express your anger?

Have you ever physically harmed someone when you were angry?

Do you smoke, drink, or use drugs of any kind?

Do you have any chronic physical conditions or illnesses?

Do you have any allergies or dietary intolerances?

Do you now have or have you ever had an STD?

When was the last time you were checked for sexually transmitted diseases?

**Why it's important:**

This set of questions is critical on multiple levels. First of all, his self-awareness of his own flaws, weaknesses, and limitations can tell you more about this person than you can possibly imagine.

Secondly, your health and safety, as well as that of your family members, should always be your top priority.

Third, it is entirely conceivable that you may be required someday to render emergency aid to your potential partner, call an ambulance, or inform an emergency room doctor of his condition or medications.

When that happens, it definitely helps to know what's wrong with him.

Finally, in the event that your relationship blossoms into a lifetime commitment, you may eventually need to accommodate his dietary needs, assist with medications, or deal with increasing levels of disability, incapacitation or even the death of your partner.

**How to interpret his answer:**

People can be notoriously secretive and touchy when it comes to their health. Tactfully seek some way to confirm what your potential Dom has told you. Also remember, that he may not actually be aware of what's wrong with him.

Addictions, anger issues, a history of violence, untreated mental illnesses, sexually transmittable diseases, and severely debilitating chronic conditions should be considered at least a yellow flag.

**What you should do about it:**

Think about what you're being told before you react to it. It can be extremely easy to blurt out something that may be interpreted as being cruel or hurtful without realizing it. Even if you *are* knowledgeable about a condition, chronic disease, or mental illness, be sure to do some additional online research to validate what you think you know before speaking.

Think long-term. Smoking, drinking, drug use, addictions, and morbid obesity are health factors that may seem like acceptable risks *now*, but have you given any thought to the consequences twenty or even fifty years down the road? Accepting a calculated risk is one thing; refusing to think about it is another thing entirely.

**My Two Cents:**

Calvin was a ladies' man, at least in the BDSM chat room that he frequented. I knew him well, or at least as well as you can know anyone when you've only text chatted online in mIRC. Each night, our chat room was typically filled with up to a hundred people at a time and had a wide following of over a two thousand members. We all eventually got quite close and one day, I suggested that we plan a real-world get-together of sorts.

After a great deal of group brainstorming, we settled on a hotel near Six Flags amusement park, Dallas, as a central location for the event. People would be flying in from all over the country for this party, even Calvin!

The women were all a-twitter at the exciting prospect of meeting this charmer of a Dominant. One of them, Robin, even offered to let him stay at her apartment in nearby Fort Worth. Since I was a close friend of Robin's, I offered to pick him up at DFW airport and take him to her place while she prepped for the party.

I met him at the airport, and was shocked to see that this internet Don Juan weighed at least 600 pounds! Not one to mince words, I greeted him with a handshake and then said, "Hi Calvin! Wow, you're a big guy! I'm guessing the flight down from Seattle must have been a tad uncomfortable for you."

He replied with a shrug, "Yeah, they made me purchase two seats and, even then, it was a pretty tight fit."

No shit, I thought. All I could do was nod and say, "Well, let's get you over to Robin's place."

At the time, I drove a sporty little Nissan. It turns out, just a little too sporty and too little. Calvin couldn't fit into the front seat of my car. I could see that the situation was embarrassing to him and at one point I seriously thought he might start crying. I finally came up with a solution to our dilemma. I reclined the front seat all the way back, so that it was practically flat, and he was then able to crawl head first over the reclined seat-back to occupy both the front and back seat like a porpoise in a helicopter sling headed for a free mackerel dinner at Sea World.

Luckily, the drive was a short one. The man smelled like a three-day old tuna sandwich. I'm rarely shy about saying what's on my mind, so I said, "Calvin, pardon me for asking, but when was the last time you bathed?"

He replied with a sheepish look, "About a year-and-a-half ago, I think. When you're as big as I am, just getting in and out of a shower can be pretty dangerous."

Again, I just nodded, not verbalizing what my brain was screaming, which was, "Ever heard of a sponge bath?"

We soon arrived at Robin's place and when she met us at the door her eyes went wide in surprise at his bulk. "Come on in and have a seat!" was about all she could manage to stammer.

Calvin waddled over to one of her dining room chairs to sit. The chair immediately disintegrated beneath him, breaking calamitously into several pieces. He sat there on the floor amongst the broken pieces of the chair for a while, weeping and muttering incoherently.

Robin seemed to be teetering on the verge of an emotional meltdown of some sort. I made a beeline for Robin's nicely stocked bar.

There *had* to be some tequila in there *somewhere*.

**Question #40:** What do you do for fun?

**Follow-up questions:**

Why was *sex* the first thing you thought about?

Do you have any hobbies?

Do you participate in any sports?

Do you watch TV or play online games?

What's your idea of a fun date?

What fun things would we do on our first date?

**Why it's important:**

Unless you want to spend the rest of your life with a partner whose idea is fun is musical flatulence or picking lint out of his navel, this question has ramifications that go well beyond small talk.

**How to interpret his answer:**

If he responds with "Do you mean sexually?" say *no*. If he *still* doesn't understand that this question isn't a sexual come-on, you've just learned pretty much all you need to know about this person.

There should be nothing hard or complicated about how to interpret his other responses to this question. Either his notion of fun makes sense to you, or it doesn't. It doesn't necessarily have to coincide with your notion of what is or isn't fun, but you should be able to at least imagine someday spending an awful lot of time around someone who does whatever it is that he does.

This is a simple question that practically everyone remembers to ask, but few people know how to derive anything useful from it.

**What you should do about it:**

Give some thought to how you might react in the future if and when he wants to involve you in his leisure time activities.

**My Two Cents:**

I'm a skydiver. Do you have a fear of heights? Then you probably won't want to jump out of a perfectly good airplane with me, but you *can* meet me on the landing zone with a cold beer.

I love trying new and exotic foods. I've eaten alligator, frog, sea turtle, kangaroo, snake, eel, raw fish, roe, and goat, just to name a few of the delicacies I've enjoyed. Are you less than adventurous when it comes to your chow? No problem. I'll bring you a tuna sandwich.

Travel calls to me. Being dropped into a culture where I don't speak the language, can't read the signs, get confused by the currency, and can't figure out what is and isn't garnish on my dinner plate is my idea of a *good time*. If the mere thought of something like that sends you into an anxiety attack, I'll take you to Disneyland instead.

I love my work and will often hyper-focus on it so intently that I forget to eat, sleep, or even acknowledge your very existence. All you have to do is remind me from time to time that I need to take a snuggle break.

Just because we both don't enjoy *everything* together, doesn't mean we can't enjoy *something* together.

**Question #41:** How do you feel about a submissive's defiant or bratty behavior?

**Follow-up questions:**

How do you react when it happens?

Do you punish it, and if so, how?

Have you ever actually had a brat submissive before?

How did that work out, or how did it end?

**Why it's important:**

Even if you are not a bratty or defiant submissive, it's important to know just how he would react if he *thought* you were. On the other hand, if you really *are* a brat, his response will tell you an awful lot about what your future relationship dynamic with this person might be like.

**How to interpret his answer:**

Just because someone thinks he'll react a certain way in any hypothetical situation, that doesn't necessarily mean that it is actually how he will react in reality. Self-delusion, unfortunately, is rampant among novice Dominants.

**What you should do about it:**

I highly recommend that you have a firm understanding of your own personal style of submission before asking this question. Otherwise, his response will be viewed through an incomplete, erroneous, or cracked prism. If you honestly don't even know what a Brat Submissive is, don't really know if you qualify as one, and have no idea why you do the things you do, how can you possibly expect to properly evaluate him as being the right or wrong Dominant for you?

As I pointed out in my previous book, a Brat Submissive is one who is generally well-behaved, but has made misbehavior, teasing, and limited kinds of defiance or disobedience an integral part of her Dominant-submissive dynamic. Preferably, this happens with the full awareness and at least the implied approval of her Dominant. When that is *not* the case, problems will arise. There is term for submissives who conduct themselves as Brats without the approval of their Dominants. We call them *phony* submissives.

**My Two Cents:**

Lolly was a Second Life submissive who was in the process of giving me a private, rather risque fashion show in that virtual 3D chat environment. As her avatar pranced and posed suggestively in a seemingly endless series of sexy outfits, she would ask, "How do you like this outfit, Sir? How about the purple one? What do you think of these nipple clamps and chains? Do you prefer me as a redhead or as a blonde?" and so on, ad nauseum.

The woman never seemed to be able to pay her real-world rent, but somehow managed to find enough real-world money to pay for her limitless supply of virtual clothing and accessories for her 3D chat avatar. I found it a little perplexing but it wasn't my circus, and not my monkey.

Personally, I've always considered these 3D avatar chat programs as sophisticated, virtual Barbie and Ken dress-up activities for adults. Even so, they can be an entertaining and mindless way to relax and stay in touch with your friends. Sometimes, they can even be useful when you are prospecting for a new Dominant, as Lolly seemed to be doing right now.

I responded to most of her questions politely but cursorily, since cartoon fashion shows aren't exactly my thing. Unfortunately, she seemed to need more than that. She began to press harder for the details of exactly what it was that I liked most or didn't like about her fashion ensembles. Finally, in response to one such inquiry, I told her in exasperation, "Lolly, I love the corset. I'm ambivalent about those stilettos. Those red eyes on your avatar, however, are really just creeping me out."

Her immediate response was shrill and plaintive. "You don't like my eyes? But I've had these red eyes for weeks, and you never said a *damn thing!!*"

I nodded and shrugged, "You never *asked.*"

These 3D chat avatars really should have cool animations where their heads explode into shards or fountains of blood start gushing from all of their facial orifices at once because if it were possible, Lolly's avatar would have been doing all of that and *more*.

She was highly pissed and barely able to articulate her sense of moral outrage in complete sentences, which I must admit, I found rather amusing. Frankly, I was just glad to have finally made my escape from that cartoon fashion show Hell masquerading as a chat program.

As she was leaving, I told her, "You know where you went wrong, don't you, Lolly? Your mistake was in asking me a question to which you were woefully unprepared to hear an honest answer."

**Question #42:** Do you punish your submissive?

**Follow-up questions:**

How do you punish your submissive?

Please tell me about the last time you had to punish a submissive.

What sorts of infractions would cause to you to feel that you must punish your submissive?

**Why it's important:**

Not all Dominants punish their submissives. Of those who do, there may be an infinite number of different ways to accomplish it. One Dominant may give you spankings, while another may ignore you for days or weeks. Still another might even release you for your transgression. The time to find out is before you make the mistake of thinking you know what the possible consequences will be.

**How to interpret his answer:**

As we've cautioned in previous sections, your first task should be to ascertain his experience and knowledge levels, so you can accurately gauge his lifestyle credibility.

Once you know that you can believe what he tells you in response to this question, then you'll need to decide whether or not you can accept the kinds of punishments (or lack thereof) that he employs.

**What you should do about it:**

Do not test your prospective Dominant's resolve to punish or not punish, as the case may be. Do not dare him to tame you, break you, train you by force, or otherwise apply any sort of discipline to you until you are absolutely certain that he is credible and that you know what is likely to happen as a result. Do not mistake patience and compassion for weakness. Do not think that just because you got away with something once, or even more often than that, that it is acceptable or that you won't be punished for it.

## My Two Cents:

"Wait!" cried April. "You're going to punish me for what I did, when Gina is allowed to get away with it without any consequences at all? Where's the fairness in that?"

"Excuse me?" I replied. "What makes you think Gina, or anyone for that matter, is allowed to disrespect me the way you just did?"

April was really angry now. "Oh, now you're *really* pissin' me off, Sir! Are you calling me a *liar?!* I have seen Gina do exactly that, last week, in fact! Why is she allowed to do it, when I am not?"

I sighed, thinking, why can't people ever be envious of doing the right thing? They see someone doing the wrong thing, and the first thing that pops into their pointy little heads is: Well, if *they* can get away with it, why shouldn't *I* be able to?

April was trying my patience. I told her, "I told you when I took you on for training that I would praise you in public, and punish you in private. How or whether I punish you is no one's business but yours and mine. That goes for Gina, as well. You may not be aware of this, but for her blatant disrespect last week, she was told to go away and not come back for two days."

"T-t-two days?" she stammered. "No... I wasn't aware of that, Sir."

"No, of course not," I replied. "That's because it was none of your damn business. Instead of learning from her mistake, you instead *envied* her. You wanted what she had which, in your misinformed mind, was the right to disrespect me without consequence. Isn't that so?"

"I... I don't know." she said, sulking. "I suppose I was envious of the privileges she always seemed to get that I was never offered. Yes, Sir."

"You saw them as privileges to be envied," I countered. "I saw them as infractions requiring disciplinary action. You didn't know that she was being punished. All you cared about was getting a piece of what you thought she had."

April nodded silently. Tears were now streaming down her face.

"Since you envy Gina so much," I said, "You can have a double helping of what she got. Come back in four days. I don't want to hear a single peep out of you until then. Goodnight, April."

**Question #43:** Do you prefer submissives or slaves?

**Follow-up questions:**

Why?

**Why it's important:**

Some people believe that a submissive's commitment to her Dominant is stronger than a slave's because the submissive chooses to be with him, whereas a slave purportedly has no choice. Others believe that a slave's commitment to her Master is the stronger because she is his property, and she knows that she cannot walk away, even if she wants to. The truth is, *both* subs and slaves have choices and both exercise those choices on a regular basis. The most important aspect of this question will be the matter of ascertaining whether your prospective Dominant's views on this matter are compatible with yours.

**How to interpret his answer:**

You should focus almost entirely on two issues: choice and property. Regardless of whether you consider yourself a sub or slave, you will need to settle these two issues.

How much choice do you have in your relationship dynamic and in your day-to-day decision-making? Are you ever allowed to tell your Dominant *no?* If not, why not? If so, under what circumstances would it be appropriate?

The issue of property is another minefield that requires careful navigation if you're going to get through it unscathed. Would you be his property? Why or why not? What does that mean? As property, could you be abused indiscriminately, loaned to others for their sexual gratification, or even sold to the highest bidder? Whose body is this and what are the limits, if there are any, to what the owner can or can't do with it?

## What you should do about it:

Do not be tempted to gloss over this question or the discussion that will surely result from it. Do take what he says seriously, especially if he considers his sub or slave to be property that he may do with as he will.

## My Two Cents:

Christine was working her way through a series of interview questions when she got to this one: "Would I be your property if you were my Dom?"

I replied, "That depends. Would you want to be?"

She looked perplexed and asked, "What's *that* supposed to mean? It's a pretty simple question. Answer yes or no. That shouldn't be difficult for a smart guy like you. Would I be your property, or not?"

"No, you would *not*," I replied, matter-of-factly. "Some of my submissives are considered my property. That is true. But it isn't because I have a one-size-fits-all policy of considering subs to be property. It's a matter of considering their wants and needs. If it pleases her to be considered my property, then I am far more likely to do so."

She chewed on that for a moment, before asking me, "Well then, why did you say you wouldn't consider *me* as your property? I haven't told you what *my* preferences are, yet."

I just shook my head. "Lady, I'm having a hard enough time just considering you a *submissive.*"

**Question #44:** Are you polyamorous?

**Follow-up questions:**

Are you poly in a theoretical sense, or do you have actual experience in poly relationships?

When, where and under what circumstances?

How and why did those relationships end?

What would you do differently, if you were to do that again?

If you consider yourself to be polyamorous, how does another partner get added to the relationship?

Would I be allowed to establish other relationships of any kind?

If you are monogamous, is your belief in monogamy based on religious values, upbringing, political views, or something else?

**Why it's important:**

There are plenty of people who will disagree with me on this, but I honestly believe that most people are either born monogamous or born polyamorous. This is usually not a problem for *either*, unless there are things going on that run counter to their nature or unless someone attempts to switch teams from mono to poly or vice versa.

**How to interpret his answer:**

This is one of those questions that can be rather tricky. The reason is the probability of self-delusion is quite high when it comes to this particular subject.

There is never a shortage of people who will swear upon a stack of bibles that they are monogamous, yet secretly wish they had multiple relationship partners. There are also many who consider themselves polyamorous in theory, but have none of the skills or experience necessary to know whether they truly *are* or to pull it off when and if they get the opportunity. If all that didn't make you wary, consider the fact that it is extremely common for misinformed people to confuse polyamory for *polyfuckery*.

In other words, when it comes to the subject of polyamory, a large number of people are just chock full of *crapola*. Some of them know that they're full of it; others are simply misinformed, self-delusional, or have no clue.

**What you should do about it:**

Be sure you know who and what *you* are before attempting to figure out whether your potential Dom is going to be compatible with that. Treat whatever he tells you on this subject with a healthy amount of skepticism.

**My Two Cents:**

Polyamory *isn't* promiscuity and it *isn't* swinging. Just because people love more than one person doesn't mean they love everyone and it definitely doesn't mean they want to bed random strangers. You don't have to *be* polyamorous to educate yourself and understand what it *is* or *isn't*.

**Question #45:** Have you ever cheated on your relationship partner?

**Follow-up questions:**

If so, what were the circumstances?

Have you ever had one of your relationship partner cheat on you?

If so, what were those circumstances?

What do you think qualifies as cheating?

Would cheating have to involve actual sex?

How about cybersex? What about phone sex? Chatting online? Flirting? Looking at porn?

**Why it's important:**

Infidelity can happen, whether you're monogamous or polyamorous. Quite often, accusations of cheating are made simply because two people can't agree on what does or doesn't constitute cheating.

Even if you've never cheated and would never even think about cheating on your partner, there's still no guarantee that you won't be accused of it.

**How to interpret his answer:**

It's rather rare for someone who cheats to casually admit to it in response to a question like this one, so do try to keep that in mind.

**What you should do about it:**

The crucial task at-hand will be to figure out where the two of you differ on what does or doesn't constitute cheating.

There are a lot of Dominants out there who would consider simply having a conversation with another Dominant as cheating. There are even some who would consider looking at porn as cheating. You may honestly believe you would never cheat on your partner, but your partner may have other ideas about what cheating means.

**My Two Cents:**

My good friend Audrey was *livid*. She'd just learned that her Dominant, Richard, had secretly been sleeping with her best friend for at least the past six months.

I let her rant and pace and hit things with her fists for about thirty minutes before expecting her to return to any semblance of calm or rationality. Then, I asked, "And how is what he did any worse than what you've been doing, sleeping with Richard's friend Joe for the last few weeks?"

"Oh sure!!" she bawled. "Take *his* side, why don't you!?"

**Question #46:** If we were in a disagreement or argument, how would you handle it?

**Follow-up questions:**

How often do you end up in arguments?

Why do you argue?

Do you like to argue?

How important is it for you to win an argument?

How do you feel when someone argues with you?

How often do you turn out to be wrong?

How do you feel when you're the one who's wrong?

How would you recommend I proceed, if I disagree with you about something?

What's the key to ending an argument with you agreeably?

**Why it's important:**

Some people are never wrong. At least, they're never wrong in their own minds. Those people can be hell to live with. Arguments aren't necessarily always a bad thing. Not knowing how to *end* one almost always is.

**How to interpret his answer:**

Trust your gut. Listen intently and attempt to read between the lines. Unfortunately, people who are never wrong will never admit to thinking that they are never wrong.

**What you should do about it:**

Try not to get into an argument about whether or not he argues. That would just be silly.

## My Two Cents:

Brenda was angry with me. "I *hate* it when you call me *stupid*, Master. I *hate hate hate* it!"

"I didn't call you stupid, babe." I replied. "What I said was, what you *did* was stupid. And it was. You know it was."

"Maybe so, Master. But I hate it when you use that word and I hate being called stupid," she said.

"Again, I never said you were stupid," I said. "We all make stupid mistakes. Smart people sometimes *do* stupid things. When they do, they learn from their mistakes and move on. How about *we* learn from this mistake and just move on?"

"The only thing I care about right *now*," she replied, "is that you stop calling me stupid. You know it triggers my anxiety. You have no idea how upset it makes me when you do that. I need you to stop. Please, Master, *just stop!*"

"Babe, I can't stop doing something that I've never done in the first place," I said. "And I'm not going to sit here and allow you continue to accuse me of doing something that I'm simply not doing at *all*."

Brenda just wasn't ready to let go of it. "But can't you see what this is doing to me? Don't you understand? Why can't you show just a little compassion? Why do you have to be such a *jerk* about this?" She was sobbing hysterically, now.

I closed my eyes and attempted to calm myself.

It took every ounce of willpower at my disposal to resist the overwhelming urge to characterize this...entire... discussion... as... incredibly...

*silly.*

**Question #47:** What do you think of slave contracts?

**Follow-up questions:**

Have you ever used one?

If so, may I see a copy of it?

If so, how did that work out for you?

**Why it's important:**

Slave contracts (the generic term for all contracts of this type) are written agreements which purport to define the rules governing a D/s relationship dynamic. Since slavery has been illegal in the United States since the end of the Civil War slave contracts, by definition, are illegal and unenforceable in any court of law.

They *can,* however, be very useful as a way to clarify expectations and intentions at the beginning of a D/s relationship. On the other hand, I have seen them used to threaten, coerce, and intimidate novice slaves and subs who were completely unaware that slave contracts are null and void in all fifty states.

**How to interpret his answer:**

There's nothing wrong with believing in or using slave contracts. As I've said, they can be useful in many ways. You should, however, listen carefully for any indication that your prospective Dominant thinks that a slave contract can be used to pressure or force you do anything against your will.

**What you should do about it:**

Consent can be revoked at any time. It doesn't matter if you've said *"yes"* a thousand times, it only takes one *"no"* to revoke your consent. Treat any discussion of using a slave contract to coerce you into doing anything you don't want to do as a red flag.

By law, any contract that requires a party to the contract to break *any* law is automatically null and void. A contract that requires someone to perform any kind of sexual acts is by definition a contract for prostitution, which is against the law in most places. A contract that refers to slavery in any way is worthless, since slavery is illegal in all fifty states. Any contract that involves a threat of bodily harm is going to be illegal because agreements made under duress are automatically deemed to be invalid.

Whatever you do, don't let anyone bamboozle you into thinking that a slave contract is a *real* contract. It *isn't*.

**My Two Cents:**

My friend Erica was at her wit's end. She'd just broken up with her Master, but he was now threatening to sue her for breach of contract. She had agreed to a slave contract several months ago but, as events progressed, she realized that he had lied to her about a great many things. Now that she had put an end to their relationship, he was attempting to use the contract to force her to accept him back as her Master.

"I can't afford a lawyer," she sobbed. "And I can't afford to travel to Florida, where he's going to file the lawsuit. I'm just completely fucked. What can I do?"

"You don't need a lawyer," I told her. "And you don't need to go to Florida, because he's not going to file a lawsuit."

"How do you *know* that?" she asked.

"First of all," I replied, "it's a rather well-known principle of the law that you are required to file lawsuits in the jurisdiction where the offense occurred and/or where the defendant lives. Otherwise, plaintiffs would always sue you in a jurisdiction so far away that you wouldn't be able to travel there to defend yourself and they'd always win by default. Second, slave contracts are unenforceable in all fifty states. That's why pimps can't use the courts to force their girls to keep whoring. Because it's illegal."

"So, what should I do now?" she asked.

"Stop taking him seriously." I replied. "Tear that ridiculous contract up and get on with your life. If he contacts you again, report him to the police as someone who is stalking and harassing you."

"I'll do that," she said. "I *owe* you one!"

I laughed. "Yes, you do!" I pointed at a random document on my desk. "It says so right there, in the contract which you never saw or signed, right after the Sex on Saturdays Clause and before the Spanking Penalties Addendum."

**Question #48:** What would your reaction be if I were to tell you that I had a sexually transmitted disease?

Important note: Ask this question *only* as appropriate and necessary. Do ***not*** ask this purely as a hypothetical question. To do so would likely serve only to generate unnecessary fear, suspicion, or contention.

**Follow-up questions:**

How much do you know about this disease?

Does it frighten you?

Have you ever known anyone who had it?

Would you like me to tell you more about it?

Are you aware that people with this condition can live fairly normal, happy lives with the proper precautions?

Does knowing this change how you feel about me?

**Why it's important:**

If this is applicable to you, then your prospective partner has a right to know and to be able to make an informed decision regarding this issue. The timing of this question is obviously going to be sensitive. It should be posed only after serious interest in you has been expressed but before any serious commitments have been made between you. Pose this question too *early* and you'll run the risk of frightening him off before he has any reason to consider the question seriously. Pose the question to him too *late* in the process, and you'll run the risk of being accused of withholding vital information. This is a delicate balancing act, indeed.

**How to interpret his answer:**

Expect him to experience a wide range of emotions upon hearing this revelation. Those emotions may include shock, dismay, disappointment, anger, sadness, compassion, frustration, or confusion.

**What you should do about it:**

As long as your dialog continues beyond the initial revelation and subsequent discussion, you should feel encouraged. If his initial reaction is difficult to read or is disappointing, consider giving him a little time to adequately digest what he has learned. Resolve to revisit the subject a day or two later.

**My Two Cents:**

Jillian, a woman I'd recently been chatting with online, had just told me that she was afflicted with genital herpes. She probably expected me to run screaming in the other direction as a result of this disclosure, but I hadn't.

She seemed a little perplexed by that. "I just wanted to tell you," she said, "before you got *too* interested in me."

"I truly appreciate the fact that you did," I replied. "It really doesn't change anything, as far as I am concerned, but thank you very much for telling me."

"It doesn't scare you?" she asked, a little incredulously.

I shrugged. "You're two thousand miles away and, at most, we've had a couple of casual online chats. There's probably about a one in a thousand chance that we'll ever meet in real life. And maybe a one in ten-thousand chance that we'll ever end up in a sexual relationship. Given those odds, I'd say worrying about catching an STD from you is probably just a little premature, wouldn't *you?*"

She tentatively agreed, and our chats continued for a time. In the end, we never *did* meet in real life. It really had nothing at *all* to do with her affliction.

She simply turned out to be *insane*.

**Question #49:** What does a collar mean to you?

**Follow-up questions:**

Please compare or contrast your thoughts on collars with your notions on marriage.

If you were to collar me, how would my collar differ from the others you've given?

Would my collar be an actual physical collar or something more symbolic?

What milestones or qualifications would be necessary before you'd offer a collar to someone?

**Why it's important:**

Collars represent different things to different people. Some view the collar as a mere acknowledgment that the two of you are connected in some way. Some see it as a way to mark their property and warn off other Dominants. Still others see it as a commitment surpassing even marriage in depth and seriousness. Major problems can develop when you and your partner can't see eye-to-eye on the meaning of your collar. If *he* sees it as a way to mark his property while *you* see it as a mere fashion accessory, you can expect choppy seas ahead.

**How to interpret his answer:**

Accept what he tells you at face value. Use analogies and comparisons to clarify any parts that need it. It is critical that you have a very clear understanding of his thinking on this matter *before* you accept his collar.

**What you should do about it:**

Evaluate what he has told you regarding his thoughts on collars, and compare them with your own collaring philosophy. If they don't mesh well, consider immediately moving on to find a more compatible prospect. I have seen submissives hang on for years, attempting to convince a prospective Dominant to change his thinking on collars. It simply isn't going to happen, any more than he could change your notions on marriage. Don't waste your precious time. You'll never get those weeks, months, or years *back*.

**My Two Cents:**

Deena decided to use the direct approach today: "When are you going to offer me your collar, Sir?"

It was a question she had managed to pose to me at least once a week for the past few months. My answer was almost always the same. "When and *if* you are ready for it, that's when."

"But how will I know when that is?" she asked. "I've been *trying* really hard to be worthy of your collar. You *know* how hard I've been trying, Sir."

I nodded. "Yes, I know you try hard. That has never been an issue. But trying isn't the same as actually doing the things which must be accomplished before you can be seriously considered. You may be trying to work through your jealousy issues, but you've been failing miserably and we both know it. You may be trying to fix your bi-polar disorder without seeing a doctor or getting medicated, but that is in direct contradiction of what I've told you needs to happen before I will even consider offering you a collar. Trying may count in pee-wee T-ball, but it just isn't going to cut it when it comes to a relationship between us."

"But *Sir*," she protested, "I wouldn't be jealous any more if I was wearing your collar. And my mood swings become magnified because of my insecurity and poor self-image. I see all these other women wanting to be yours, and it just makes me that much more miserable and moody. But being yours would help to fix that!"

"I'm sorry, but you're just flat-out wrong on this," I replied. "Slapping a collar on an already messed-up submissive only makes things worse, not better. Trust me on this. This ain't my first rodeo."

"I just know that I'd be better able to handle my jealousy and mood swings if I was collared to you." she countered. "I just *know* it!"

I shook my head. "We are *not* going to test that little hypothesis out. Would you just hand someone your car keys and tell them to go out and learn to drive? No, you wouldn't. Learn to drive first and then you can borrow my car keys. Until then, trying is a good thing. It's a very good thing. But trying alone isn't going to cut it. Like Yoda says: Do, or do not. There is no try."

**Question #50:** To what degree should I hold you responsible for my wants, needs, or desires not being considered or fulfilled?

**Follow-up questions:**

Are you concerned only about my sexual, BDSM, or D/s needs?

Which of my needs are you least concerned with or least responsible for?

Where do your responsibilities end?

What will be the remedy when my wants and needs aren't being met by you?

**Why it's important:**

Shit happens. The best-laid plans of Dominants and submissives will oft go awry. When they *do*, what's your plan?

**How to interpret his answer:**

There shouldn't be a lot of interpretation necessary here, but do listen carefully for any attempt to sidestep or tap-dance around the notion that he should be held accountable for what he does or doesn't accomplish in your relationship.

**What you should do about it:**

"Not my problem" shouldn't be something you ever have to hear in any real-world full-time D/s relationship. Once you enter into such a relationship with a Dominant, it's your job to hold him accountable to the extent that he has agreed to be held accountable. Similarly, it's his job to hold you accountable to the degree that you've agreed to be held accountable.

If you skipped over this particular discussion when you should have been working out some sort of an agreement regarding those little details, you're both screwed.

**My Two Cents:**

In a nutshell, Dominants like feeling responsible for what happens. Submissives like holding Dominants responsible for what happens. But the *truth* is you're *both* responsible for what happens in your relationship.

Worrying about who should be blamed when things go wrong is a terrible waste of emotional energy and has never solved a damn thing.

**Question #51:** Have you ever collared a submissive or slave before?

**Follow-up questions:**

Was it online or real-life?

How long did that collar last?

What were the circumstances of his or her release?

What other circumstances would be possible reasons for releasing submissive or slave?

**Why it's important:**

As has been the case is many of the other questions that we've covered to this point, it's critical that you figure out just how much of his knowledge, experience, and lifestyle philosophy is theoretical. There's an old joke that's been going around for as long as I can remember that goes, "I used to have five scientific theories on how to best raise happy, healthy, well-adjusted children. Now, I have five kids, and no theories."

The same sort of thing happens when a Dominant collars a submissive for the first time or, for that matter, the first few times. All those notions you had before the collar suddenly go out the window the moment they butt up against cold, hard reality. In the army, we had a saying. No battle plan ever survives first contact with the enemy.

**How to interpret his answer:**

Your first priority is to determine whether your prospective Dominant is speaking from experience or from his fertile imagination. Either way, your next priority is to decide whether you are comfortable with his purported reasons for collaring or releasing subs. To make this a little easier, take some of his assertions and mentally substitute the word "marriage" for "collar." You may end up with something like, "I've been married eight times and most of them only lasted about a week or two."

**What you should do about it:**

If he seems credible and compatible, explore further the possibility of a collar in the future. If he is neither credible nor compatible with you, you don't really need *me* to tell you what to do about it, do you?

**My Two Cents:**

If you have been reading this book from the beginning, you're probably starting to get the idea that I have collared hundreds of submissives in the course of my thirty-seven years in this lifestyle. I have *not*.

I really don't know exactly how many there have been, but my best guess would be perhaps a couple dozen in the course of 37 years, if you want to count training collars and such in addition to the formal relationship collars. I've also been married a few times. More than a few times, if you want to count common-law marriages and cohabitations.

Another thing that contributes to this illusion of quantity over quality is the fact that I often change the names of the people I'm writing about. Sometimes, I do it to spare them embarrassment or unnecessary attention. Other times, I'll do it so it doesn't seem as though all of my stories are about the same individuals, again and again and again.

It isn't at all unusual for me to tell one of my submissives, "Hey, sweetie! Remember that time when we did this, that, or the other thing? Well, I just wrote a little story about it for the book and this time, your name is *Agatha!* Why don't you give it a quick read and tell me what you think?"

My partners are all wonderful and unique individuals, each as different as can be. But when it comes to this sort of thing, their responses are invariably identical. *"Ewww!* Master!! Agatha? Seriously? Why *Agatha? Yuckkk!"*

Nevertheless, I do get a great deal of enjoyment from immortalizing the submissives I love in my writing. It gives me a chance to share with the rest of the world the many incredible things that I see in them. Sometimes, it's their strength, beauty, intelligence, compassion, resourcefulness, or wonderful sense of service and submission. Other times, it's their all-too-human weaknesses, tragic flaws, hard-headedness, silly little mistakes, or deep-rooted insecurities. Regardless, I loved them *all* and there will always be a place in my heart for each of them... even the ones who cursed me on their way out the door.

I write about them not because I want to cause any of them any amount of emotional distress, but because they are and always will be a part of me, and because I want *you* to learn from *our* mistakes without having to make all of those very same mistakes on your own. And yes, I said *our* mistakes.

I *am* willing to share responsibility for much of what has gone wrong in my previous relationships. As I've said before, however, I don't believe that assigning and dwelling on blame solves much of anything.

I can't promise anyone that I love that she'll never see herself in one of my books. About the best I can do is promise her that I won't call her *Agatha.*

**Question #52:** Would you want to manage my contacts and friendships?

**Follow-up questions:**

Would that include my online friends and acquaintances?

Would that include my real-life friends?

What sorts of things would cause you to ask me to break off a friendship?

**Why it's important:**

You may find this surprising, but this question addresses a topic that is one of the most common bones of contention in D/s relationships. *Some* Dominants attempt to assuage their own insecurities by attempting to govern every aspect of your social life. As one might imagine, most people have never experienced anything quite so controlling and don't react well to such things as being told that they must cut all ties to their friends or family members, allow your emails and texts to be read, and have all of your phone calls monitored. It is typically a technique used by insecure Doms with severe jealousy issues or phony Doms to isolate you from anyone who might tell you that they are clueless.

**How to interpret his answer:**

This will be one of those questions that will require a great deal of discussion before you can finally arrive at any semblance of the truth. It's extremely rare that anyone will voluntarily admit to being clingy and insecure, especially if he thinks he's a Dominant or is pretending to be one. Additionally, it's a common thing for the people with the most severe jealousy issues to make an annoying habit of blaming everyone but themselves for the havoc that it wreaks in their relationships.

**What you should do about it:**

A Dominant who is competent, socially adept, and confident will have no problem with his submissives going places and doing things with friends, making and taking phone calls or texts, or spending occasional time alone. If he says he does or demonstrates that that he might, consider that a red flag.

**My Two Cents:**

I require strangers who want to add my submissive as a friend on Facebook, Fetlife, or any other social media sites to contact me first. I don't make them jump through any hoops or do anything special. All they have to do is contact me and say, "Would it be all right if I added Evelyn as a friend?" Ninety-nine percent of the time I automatically say *yes,* unless I already know that person to be a *twat-waffle*. It's simply a little ritual that makes my girls feel safer and reassures me that the stranger is at least willing to acknowledge that she is owned before he starts stalking her.

One guy named *Redbeard* just didn't seem to get it, though. When my submissive Evelyn explained to him that he'd have to contact me before she would accept his friend request, his first reaction was to scold and insult her.

"What??" he messaged back. "This is America, not some fucking communist country where you have to get permission to accept my friend request, you *dumb cunt!"*

Evelyn was both shocked and amused by his response and showed me the message. I laughed and told her if he didn't want to contact me, well then, I'll contact *him!*

"Dear Mr. Redbeard," I wrote. "Thank you for your thoroughly entertaining treatise on the relative merits of post-industrial-age communism as it pertains to random, unsolicited Fetlife friend requests. Please allow me to clarify the procedure to you in terms that even a knuckle-dragging, mouth-breathing twat-waffle like yourself should be able to understand. Evelyn does not need to get my permission to friend anyone. She's a grown woman and I trust her judgment implicitly. You, on the other hand, remind me of something I've had to scrape off the bottom of my shoe. Eve isn't the one who needs permission. *You* are, Einstein. As for calling her a dumb cunt, I suggest we simply agree to disagree on that matter until I see you again, at which time I will just *beat* a proper apology out of you. Sincerely, Michael Makai."

**Question #53:** What kinds of collars do you employ?

**Follow-up questions:**

Do you believe in Collars of Consideration?

Do you believe in Training Collars?

Do you believe in Formal Collars?

Do you believe in using Day Collars?

What do you think would be the biggest change in our dynamic if I were collared to you?

**Why it's important:**

Not everyone in the lifestyle embraces the practice of collaring and even those who do may have widely differing beliefs about what it all means. This topic becomes much more important if you have strong notions about it yourself. If you don't believe in the use of training collars, for example, being asked to wear one could become a major sticking point in your budding relationship.

**How to interpret his answer:**

Listen carefully to his response and view it as a statement of preference. If, for example, he says that he uses collars of consideration, interpret it as saying he prefers to use collars of consideration. You would have a say in the matter, and if that sort of collar isn't something you want, this is a good time to let him know that. Every collar, no matter what type of collar it may be, is a symbol of a mutual agreement.

**What you should do about it:**

Once you feel you have a good understanding of your prospective Dom's collaring philosophy, use this discussion as a chance to tell him what your thoughts on collars are, and to reach some common understanding, if not agreement on what would or would not work for the two of you when and if the time comes.

Do *not* fall into the trap of thinking that this discussion is an *offer* of a collar, or that it should necessarily *lead* to an offer of a collar. Just because you're talking about collars, that doesn't mean someone is *getting* one.

**My Two Cents:**

I get asked about collars quite often. I'm an old-school Dominant, which means that I tend to view a collar as a very serious commitment that surpasses even marriage in some ways. My preference has always been a poly Dom/sub dynamic, but most of my relationships tend to have attributes that are somewhat characteristic of a typical Master/slave relationship dynamic. Consequently, I get asked a ton of questions on the topic of collars.

My philosophy is often atypical of other Dominants in the lifestyle, so take that for what it's worth. BDSM is not a religion and I am not its high priest. What works for me may not work for you, and vice versa. If you find what I've written useful, awesome possum! If not, life goes on and I'll get over it.

Personally, I *don't* think collars of consideration are a good idea. For those who may not be aware of what a collar of consideration is, it is a collar offered to a submissive that signifies and announces to the world that she is being considered for a formal collar. The submissive is typically expected to stop shopping around for a Dom while she is under consideration and the Dominant is expected to evaluate her suitability and explain what she may have to do to prove herself worthy of a formal collar. Either party can walk away from this collar agreement at any time, without explanation.

Just imagine how this would work for a vanilla couple. You go out with a prospective boyfriend and he offers you a ring on your first date which means that he is thinking about making you his fiancée. Afterwards, you show everyone your new ring and tell them, "This symbolizes our commitment to think about getting engaged!"

You're very excited, your girlfriends are all very excited, and your family thinks you're certifiably *nuts*. After a few weeks of this, your prospect suddenly tells you that he has decided that he's no longer thinking about it, and with no explanation whatsoever, he summarily asks for his ring back. You figure, okay, maybe this guy is just a jerk. But then it happens again with the next guy, and again with the next one as well.

*That's* what it's like for most of the submissives and slaves who accept collars of consideration and *that's* why I don't like them.

**Question #54:** If I was collared to you and you felt that you had to release me, how would you do it?

**Follow-up questions:**

Have you ever had to release a sub in the past?

If so, how did you go about it?

What were the consequences to each of you, if any?

If I wanted to be released from my collar at some point in the future, how should I go about it?

**Why it's important:**

Nothing lasts forever. *Nothing.*

**How to interpret his answer:**

Listen to his answer without judgment and clarify anything that you don't fully understand. As usual, make an attempt to determine how much of his response is purely theoretical and how much is the result of practiced application.

**What you should do about it:**

If he tries to tell you that it will never happen, you should interpret that as a sign that he may be dangerously naive about the real odds of success in any relationship. If he considers release a possibility, but has never actually given it any thought, consider it an indicator of over-optimism and poor contingency planning. If he does have a realistic notion of how it ought to be handled, be thankful. If he sounds like he has done it a thousand times, *be wary.*

**My Two Cents:**

In my world, there are just two ways to get yourself released: You can do it accidentally or you can do it on-purpose. Of the two, on-purpose is usually the better option.

The following is an example of how it can happen accidentally:

"Master, why didn't you tell me about your lunch date today with Daisy?" asked Jennifer, plaintively. "You *know* I like to be kept informed about such things!"

"I *did* tell you about it," I replied. "I told you just now, as soon as I walked in the front door. What, exactly, were you hoping for? A running commentary in real-time, as it was happening? That would just be stupid."

She had severe anxiety issues and I suffered from chronic *snark*; not a good mix at *all*. She was starting to get very agitated and the pitch of her voice suddenly became shrill. "Oh! So now I'm stupid, am I? Your sarcasm is bad enough; you skipped your usual sarcasm and went right to being insulting and condescending. Master, you *know* that's not what I meant. Just once, I would like to see just a little compassion from you. Instead of considering the gut-wrenching anxiety I go through every time you refuse to tell me what I need to know when I need to know it, you insult me. It's like a slap in the face and I just can't take it any longer!"

I sighed, realizing in that moment that I'd inadvertently set her off on one of her anxiety-laden emotional death-spirals. When she got that way, there was nothing you could say or do that would calm her down or return her to rationality.

"Look, babe," I told her, "I'm very sorry you feel that I've been insulting or condescending. I can assure you that that was never my intent. But I also need you to understand that I can't let your anxiety issues run my life. I told you in the beginning that I would do my best to understand it and adapt, but I also told you that I wasn't going to change who or what I was in order to accommodate it. I know you're upset and, frankly, I'm getting a little upset too. How about we take a day or two to cool down a bit, and then we'll discuss it when we can do so calmly, without attacking each other?"

She just couldn't let it go. "Oh, *now* I'm *attacking* you?? *Jesus*, Master, why do you have to be so mean-spirited? A *real* Dominant would show some fucking compassion! You think we need a couple days to cool off? You know what? I'm going to need a hell of a lot more than that! I'm going to need a couple weeks. Even better, how about a couple *months?* Maybe by then, you can learn how not to be such a *jerk!"*

"Two months it *is*, then," I replied. "Be careful what you ask for, babe. You're about to get it. We'll talk again in two months, and not a moment sooner. *Goodnight.*"

We never did have that talk.

Conversely, here's an example of how a release is done on-purpose:

"Master, it pains me to have to say this because I care for you deeply, but I can no longer devote the necessary time and attention to this relationship that you deserve. I now have other priorities and think I may wish to explore the possibility of a relationship with someone else. I hope we will always be close, but will understand if that will be difficult for you. May I please be released?"

# Chapter 3: Before a Collar

There is often a small window of opportunity that exists between a first meeting and a collaring that you should definitely take advantage of to ask a few *more* questions. These questions focus on the next step in your developing relationship, which may or may not involve a collar. Regardless, once you have met in real-life, your focus shifts from whether meeting is a good idea at all to whether or not the two of you should proceed on to the next step, which may include a committed relationship of some kind.

Whether that relationship features a collar or *not,* there will always be a host of important issues which must be considered. Those issues include complicated matters such as children, finances, careers, household pets, friends and family, property, and lines of authority. If you have successfully interviewed your prospective Dominant during the pre-meet phase of your developing relationship, these questions will be easy in comparison. If, on the other hand, you've skipped over much of that process, these questions will be much more difficult. It's a little like skipping over the "let's do lunch" question, and jumping right to the "who pays the tab" one. Awkward *and* painful.

There is one more very important thing you should be keeping top-of-mind during this phase of getting to know your prospective Dominant. If you are smart, you will *not* have already made the decision to accept a collar before actually meeting your Dom.

I realize the temptation is great to accept a collar early in the process and that it helps you to muster up the courage needed to actually meet him face to face, especially if he attempts to make that decision for you. I will admit that I've made this mistake myself a few times, but let there be no doubt about it... it *was* a mistake.

Here's what you must consider: A collar can be a lifetime commitment that surpasses even marriage in its gravitas and consequences. Would you marry someone without even meeting him *once?*

**Question #55:** Now that you've met me, was I what you expected?

**Follow-up questions:**

If not, what were you expecting?

If not, why were you expecting that?

If not, were you surprised or disappointed?

Now that we have met, has your thinking changed at all regarding our potential relationship?

Would you like to know how you compared with my expectations?

If you could do it all over again, what would you change regarding how we met and how things went for us?

**Why it's important:**

Expectation can be a double-edged sword that both excites and motivates you in the early stages of this process, but also often disappoints and demotivates you when the expectation turns out to be an unrealistic fantasy based more upon wishful thinking than reality. Sometimes, the expectation can be *so* detached from the facts that coming face-to-face with reality becomes a jarring and possibly catastrophic experience.

**How to interpret his answer:**

This question is always going to be one that is incredibly difficult to discuss rationally and do it in a way that doesn't hurt someone's feelings. It is simply human nature to present yourself in the best possible light to any prospective partner. If you have two photos and one of them makes you look sexier, fitter, healthier, or happier than the other it shouldn't take a rocket scientist to figure out which one you're going to show to people. Unrealistic expectations are also a part of human nature. We don't fantasize about the things we *don't* want and *aren't* interested in.

**What you should do about it:**

Hope may spring eternal in our hearts and minds, but it makes for a lousy strategy for success when it comes to finding the right partner in this lifestyle. Don't just sit around hoping for someone who has the qualities you seek in a mate. You should be actively seeking out those qualities in a prospective Dominant and doing whatever you can to verify that what you think you know about that person bears at least some resemblance to reality.

**My Two Cents:**

As I've no doubt mentioned before, I'm a short, middle-aged, geeky, half-Asian know-it-all who works in his pajamas and can barely pay the rent. I'm also hard-headed enough that I absolutely refuse to see the connection between those last two items.

Whenever someone looks at my online profiles, they will *always* see a photo of the real me. Why don't I just do what most people do and post something more anonymous? I do it because I can. I am a BDSM writer and educator. At this stage of my life, no one is going to fire me from my job or give me a poor performance review because of it. I also do it because I dislike having to disappoint someone who may have unrealistic expectations or misconceptions about who and what I am. By putting my photo right out front, I can avoid a lot of misunderstandings regarding my physical appearance, at least.

If you don't like geeky, short, half-Asian Dominants, just *move along...*

Nothin' to see here, folks!

**Question #56:** What is your "Prime Directive" or the one rule that overrides all the other rules?

**Follow-up questions:**

What makes that particular rule so important?

How did you arrive at the decision to make this rule your Prime Directive?

What happens when the Prime Directive is violated?

Can you tell me about the last time this was an issue for you and your partner?

If you had to come up with a full "Ten Commandments" that your submissive or slave would have to follow, what do you think they would be?

**Why it's important:**

Having *some* notion of what the rules may be once you are collared is a *good thing*.

**How to interpret his answer:**

You've posed this question as a hypothetical one, but you should remember this: If this Prime Directive has been in effect throughout *all* of his previous D/s relationships then it's practically a given that you, too, will eventually fall under its purview when your relationship progresses beyond the courting stage.

**What you should do about it:**

As you discuss this topic, be on the lookout for any tendency on his part to make up rules simply for the sake of having rules. Similarly, avoid pressuring him for rules that are unnecessary or impractical just because you think you should have some. That never ends well.

As your relationship develops over time, it is usually best to come up with rules as needed in response to real needs, not imaginary ones. Each time a new rule is added to your list, it should be discussed and mutually agreed upon, with special attention devoted to the real intent of the rule.

You should both do your best to avoid fuzzy language, weasel-words, euphemisms, loopholes, and emotionally-charged verbiage that could turn out to be problematic in the future. A rule like *"Don't be a cunt"* will probably cause more problems than it will solve. A rule that forbids you from "playing" with others could be interpreted to mean just about anything. Rules that make you responsible for someone else's happiness or emotional state are ridiculously unrealistic, since no one can control another person's feelings.

Your goal should be to agree upon real, enforceable rules to address real, solvable problems.

**My Two Cents:**

My friend Regina was very excited about the most recent progress that Randy, her novice Dominant, was making in the course of his training under the mentorship of a mutual friend and Dom experienced in the lifestyle. She told me,

"His mentor explained the need for some rules in our relationship, so I directed him to come up with a list of rules for me!"

I nodded, just a little bemused. "You directed Randy to do that, did you?" I asked, with a grin. I knew Randy quite well and frankly, I found the notion comical.

She laughed and replied, "Oh, I don't need your standard lecture on topping from the bottom. I know that that's what I am doing, but there's no other way. If he's going to become the Dom that I need him to be, then I'm going to have to tell him what to do."

"Is that so?" I asked, chuckling and shaking my head. "You really don't see the irony in any of that, do you? Treating him like a subbie is going to turn into an epic train wreck. Mark my words. That way, when it happens, I can tell you I told you so," I said. "Now, tell me about these rules."

She began to read from her list. "I have to journal for him daily. I have to meet him at the front door, naked and on my knees, each day when he comes home from work. I have to wear my stainless-steel collar twenty-four seven. I'm not allowed to play with any other Doms..."

"Randy is working double shifts, "I said. "When will he have time to read and comment on your journals?"

"I'll make sure he finds the time," she replied.

"Okay," I said, "and how will you meet him at the front door naked and on your knees every day? You have two young kids in the house."

"Well, obviously we'll only do that when the kids are already in bed and asleep," she explained.

"And didn't you just start a new job at the hospital?" I asked. "How are they going to feel about you wearing a steel collar to work?"

She shrugged. "I guess we'll find out," she replied.

I shook my head, and continued, "And what's this about not playing with other Doms? What, exactly, does *playing* mean? Does that mean no sex? No BDSM scenes? No sharing Snapchat pics of your tits? No coffee at Starbucks? What?"

"Hmmm," she said, pondering the implications. "I'm going to have to get back to you on that one!"

A month later, I asked Regina about Randy's training and about her new rules. She admitted that life had gotten in the way and that she had not been able to comply with a single one of her new rules. I asked her how Randy felt about that.

She laughed and said, "He's been so busy at work and so exhausted when he gets home, he's never even bothered to check to see if I was following the rules! So, I got over!"

Right, I thought, silently shaking my head... because directing your Dom to implement a list of impossible tasks and then taking pride in *getting over* on him should be the goal of *every* good D/s relationship?

**Question #57:** Where would your authority end?

**Follow-up questions:**

Would I be expected to let you tell me how to raise my kids? Does that include telling me how to discipline them, or disciplining them yourself?

Would I be expected to let you manage my paycheck, finances, and assets?

Would I be expected to let you have a say in my future career choices?

Would I be allowed any veto power in the decisions that are made?

If so, how would that happen?

**Why it's important:**

Frankly, if I need to explain to you what makes this particular set of questions important, you have bigger problems than anything this book can possibly help you with.

**How to interpret his answer:**

An experienced and knowledgeable Dominant will know not only his own limitations; he also knows that you may have some of your own, as well. We're not talking about kink limits, here. We're talking about the limits to just how impactful your D/s relationship and lifestyle is on your day-to-day existence. Most people tend to compartmentalize their lives in order to reduce the effects that their fetish lifestyle may have on the other areas of their lives where it might be considered inappropriate or not worth the hassle.

This on-going balancing act of integrating when you can, yet compartmentalizing when it is necessary, is a challenge that faces nearly all BDSM lifestylers. Anyone who seems completely oblivious to it or dismisses the importance of at least discussing the subject with you is not worth your time.

**What you should do about it:**

As has been the case with many of the preceding questions in this book, it's very important that you already have a good idea of what your own preferences on this subject are before engaging him on this topic. Even so, you might want to keep an open mind to possibilities that you may not have ever considered before.

We've all known that single mom who viscerally rejected the idea that *anyone* but her would ever be allowed to discipline her kids. Then, she marries that *one guy* that her kids actually respect and listen to and suddenly her mind is changed. You just never know what the future may hold.

Assign a yellow flag if your prospective Dominant appears to be a little oblivious to the subject at first. It's entirely possible that he simply hasn't given it much thought until now. If he goes on to seriously consider the issue and engages you in a meaningful discussion about it, then you're at least on the right track.

If your prospective Dominant discusses the issue with you, but then goes on to dismiss your preferences as being unimportant, irrelevant, or a challenge, you should toss a red flag and move on to the next candidate.

**My Two Cents:**

Before she moved to Texas with her two kids to be with me, my submissive JoAnne and I discussed the subject of child discipline, but the talks had been rather unproductive and typically ended with, "Let's cross that bridge when we get to it." Then, suddenly they were here, and there was the bridge, ready to be crossed.

I've never been a big fan of spankings, at least for children. I always reserved those for my submissives and, even then, only as a reward; not a punishment.

JoAnne's kids, 8-year old Sean and 10-year old Hailey, had learned long ago how to push Mom's buttons. They knew *exactly* how hard they had to push before she would either give up and let them have their way, or send them to their rooms. Their rooms were chock-full of toys, games, and electronics, which meant that being sent there was practically the next best thing to a trip to Disneyland. The icing on the cake for them was the fact that there was no way you could do your daily chores while you were in there!

They had figured out that there were really only two possible outcomes when it came to Mom's discipline. She would either give them what they wanted or she would send them to video game heaven for the rest of the day. It was a win-win scenario any way you sliced it. But now, I had become the new wild-card in that scenario.

Once we got them moved in, I took a few weeks to simply observe how JoAnne disciplined, paying special attention to how the kids reacted to her style of discipline. It soon became readily apparent to me what changes needed to be made, and we sat down to have a long talk about it. I asked if she would be okay with trying something just a little different and she said she would, as long as it didn't involve beatings or feeding them to wild animals.

It wasn't long before we got a chance to try our new strategy out. Sean was blatantly disrespectful to his Mom and when he got called on it, he just stood there, grinning. Obviously, he fully expected the result to be an afternoon spent playing video games in his room. He was *wrong*.

JoAnne told him, "Sean, I am done trying to discipline you. Obviously, this is not working. So from now on, when you need to be disciplined, Mike is going to be the one who does it."

The look on her son's face revealed his sudden terrible realization that he'd made a serious miscalculation about the possible outcomes to this particular scenario. Instead of sending him to his room, I led him out the front door to an uncomfortable-looking metal bench on the front porch. I told him to sit and stay right there for the next thirty minutes, and said if he gave us any guff about it, we'd make it an hour.

"Can I at least get my PSP game or a book to help pass the time?" he asked, with suddenly sad, puppy dog eyes.

I laughed out loud and replied, "No, Sean, you may *not*. This is *supposed* to be boring as crap; hopefully, enough so that you'll want to avoid it in the future. Oh, and every time you ask us if your thirty minutes is up yet, we're just going to add another ten minutes to your time. You might just end up spending all night out here!" I smiled and winked at him as I turned to go back into the house.

The kids absolutely hated spending time out on the front porch. As a result, their behavior improved dramatically in the course of the following months. JoAnne and I considered this a rare win and were relieved that we hadn't had to resort to feeding them to the bears.

# Chapter 4: After the Collar

Once you have accepted a collar from your Dominant, the process isn't over, by any stretch of the imagination. Your questions simply shift their focus once again, this time to the daily task of maintaining and improving your existing relationship. The day you stop working on these goals will likely be the beginning of the end of your relationship, and I'm guessing you don't want to go there.

Every collared relationship dynamic is going to be unique, but they should all share a certain level of respect and protocol. Please keep this in mind as you continue asking questions to your Dominant to better understand what is really going on in your relationship. The tone and underlying assumptions behind your questions should continue to be respectful and deferential. Sometimes, a question, even a *good* question, can be posed the wrong way, at the wrong time, or for the wrong reasons.

Sometimes, the question you want to ask is going to be more about your own insecurities or feelings of unworthiness than it is about your Dominant or his thinking. Do try to exercise a high level of self-awareness in the continuing process of querying your Dom. Before you blurt out a question, take a moment to ask yourself why this particular question seems important to you at this particular moment in time. Even though the question in your head may *seem* like the most important thing in the world at that moment in time, chances are pretty good that no earth-shattering catastrophe will ensue if you just sleep on it for one night before asking it.

If the answer to *why* you're asking the question turns out to be because you are feeling a momentary pang of insecurity or because you're a little hormonal today, taking one more night to sleep on it before asking might not be a bad idea, either.

It also never hurts to put a bit of a positive spin on your questions. It can certainly help to avoid misunderstandings if your Dominant is able to frame your question in the proper context.

Remember, your acceptance of a collar shouldn't give you a sense of having reached your destination. It should, instead, represent a commitment to embark upon the first steps of your new journey, *together*.

**Question #58:** Am I your property?

**Follow-up questions:**

If so, to what extent am I your property, and how does this affect our day-to-day lives and relationship dynamic?

If I am your property, is all of my property also your property? Is property allowed to own property?

If I am not your property, what is your thinking in general on the subject of D/s partners as property?

If I am your property, can I be intentionally damaged, lent out, or sold?

**Why it's important:**

Depending on your own thoughts and feelings regarding the notion of treating a partner as property, this topic may or may not hold much importance to you. Regardless, it is still going to be a good idea to find a partner whose views tend to agree with yours on this.

**How to interpret his answer:**

Just as I've cautioned you previously, your first order of business when it comes to interpreting his answer should be to separate the theoretical from the practical. It's easy for people to say they consider their subs or slaves to be their property. It's another thing entirely to see that philosophy put into action in real life.

**What you should do about it:**

If you don't want to be treated like a piece of property, then you should avoid choosing a Dominant whose stated intent is to do just that. Conversely, if you do want to be treated like his property, don't choose a Dom who is repelled by the notion.

This happens to be one of those issues where you are highly unlikely to change his opinion at any point in any future relationship. That means you should take what he tells you now at face value and avoid the trap of believing that you'll be able to convert him to your way of thinking later.

**My Two Cents:**

"How did you skin your knee?" I asked, as Nicole walked up to our table in Starbucks.

Nicole cast her eyes downward and said, "I was excited to see you, and so I was running across the parking lot in my high heels and tripped. But... it's not too bad and it doesn't hurt much, so it's not a problem."

I shook my head. "I'm sorry, but you're wrong, babe. It *is* a problem and here's why it's a problem. You belong to *me*, do you not? That means you just lacerated *my* knee as a result of your unthinking carelessness with *my* property. From now on, you need to take better care of *my* stuff. Are we clear on this?"

She nodded and replied, "Yes, Master."

**Question #59:** Would you like me to journal for you?

**Follow-up questions:**

If so, should I journal daily, weekly, or monthly?

Is there something in particular you'd like me to address in my journals?

Would my journals be private, for your eyes only?

Where and how would you like me to journal?

**Why it's important:**

A Dominant should be kept informed not only of everything that his submissive is doing but, to the greatest extent possible, what she is thinking and feeling, too. A Dom cannot make good decisions if he is uninformed. He cannot fulfill your desires if he has no idea what will make you happy. Unfortunately, knowing what is going on inside of your head is one of those things that is always far easier said than accomplished. Journaling is one way to make this difficult task a little easier for everyone involved.

**How to interpret his answer:**

If your prospective Dominant is unfamiliar with the idea of having a submissive communicate her thoughts by journaling, tactfully explain that it's like having a diary that he can read any time he wants to, and that it can help to establish better communication between the two of you.

You may find that journaling helps *you* to sort through your thoughts and feelings, and may even provide you a way to look back at what you were thinking at a specific point in the past. It's a great way to see just how far you've come in your knowledge, experience, and training.

**What you should do about it:**

If your prospective Dom sees the potential benefits of journaling and is agreeable to having you give it a try, look into one of the many online diaries or journaling web sites available for that sort of thing. One of the websites that I recommend highly is LiveJournal.com. Just be sure to adjust your account settings so your journal entries don't become viewable by the general public.

**My Two Cents:**

"Marie, why haven't you been keeping up with your journals?" I asked, sternly.

Marie seemed surprised by my question and stammered, "I... I didn't think you *cared* about it any longer! It's been weeks since you commented on any of my journal entries. I thought that it didn't really matter to you any longer!"

I shook my head. "My directive to you was that you should journal each day. I told you that you should do this, even if you felt that you had nothing to say. In those cases, I said that you should simply create a journal entry stating that you had nothing to say. Did I not?"

She nodded and meekly replied, "Yes, Sir. You did."

I pressed on. "I didn't tell you to journal daily, but only if I comment on your entries. I likewise didn't tell you to journal daily, but only until you think it's no longer important or until you think I've stopped paying attention. Were any of those loopholes part of my directive to you?"

She silently shook her head no. I continued, "You told me three months ago that you were willing to do whatever it takes to prove yourself worthy of my collar. I asked you to journal daily for me; a rather simple task, frankly. Yet in the course of the last ninety days there have been just forty-six journal entries. That is *unacceptable.*"

"Oh my god, Sir!" she gasped, "I didn't realize you were *serious!* I mean, you never said anything to me about it when I missed a day or two, so I just assumed you no longer cared about it."

"Then you assumed wrong," I said. "My intent in giving you that task was to help me to get to know what was going on inside of your head. But there were several other reasons for it, as well. I wanted to see if you'd do it even when you thought I wasn't paying attention or when you thought I didn't care. I wanted to see if you would follow my instructions to the letter or interpret them in your own way. I wanted to see if you took what I said seriously. You know, you've been asking me about when your training would start? Well, babe, it started 3 months ago, and journaling was lesson number one. So, you tell *me*. How well do you think you did? What grade should I give you?"

"Ohhhh, *crap.*" was all she could manage to say.

**Question #60:** What things may or may I not disclose to others about you or about our relationship?

**Follow-up questions:**

Please tell me what I absolutely must not tell others about you, and why.

Please tell me what I absolutely must not tell others about myself, and why.

How should I characterize our relationship to others?

**Why it's important:**

It's important because loose lips sometimes do, in fact, sink ships. I have seen seemingly strong and healthy relationships disintegrate in an instant when the wrong information was passed along to the wrong people. Whether it is done purposefully or inadvertently, the end results can be equally catastrophic.

**How to interpret his answer:**

Take his response to this question very, very seriously. You may be tempted to scoff at his apparent paranoia or dismiss his reasoning for whatever he tells you here. Do *not* succumb to that temptation. He may have some very good reasons for his preference which you may not be privy to.

**What you should do about it:**

Follow his instructions regarding what you may or may not disclose to the letter, regardless of whether or not you understand or agree with them. Every person in this lifestyle deserves to have his or her privacy respected. No one should have to live in fear of losing their job, losing their children, or being outed unnecessarily just because someone doesn't know when to keep their mouth shut. The fact that he is your Dominant and deserves your loyalty makes this principle all the more sacrosanct.

**My Two Cents:**

"Be careful what you post online," I told the classroom full of bank employees as the class drew to a close. "If you're going to post pictures of yourself snorting cocaine on your Facebook page, we're going to have to fire you. That's just the way it is. Please exercise good judgment when it comes to that sort of thing."

This *wasn't* a hypothetical scenario. We'd just had to fire a bank teller for doing exactly that. As a result, the bank's exasperated CEO had called me into his office and told me, "Mike, I want you to schedule a mandatory training session for all employees for next Saturday. You teach the class. Explain to them that once they put that stuff out there on the Internet, it never goes away. We have an obligation to distance ourselves from anyone whose actions might reflect poorly upon this institution."

At the end of the class, most of the employees filed out of the building, got into their cars, and went back home to their families. Tasha, a twenty-year old who worked in the bank's lending department, went instead to her office. She was incensed. She didn't like being told what she could and couldn't post on her Facebook page. After all, it was her personal business. What right did these ass-hats have, poking their noses into things that didn't concern them? Fucking hypocrites, all of them! Let's just see *how* hypocritical.

She googled me and found some photographs that a former submissive had posted on the internet. The photos had been taken about a year earlier at one of those very rare dungeon parties where taking photographs *was* allowed. Even so, everyone had been told, "You may take pictures only with the expressed permission of the person you're photographing, but you may *not* share them."

Apparently, the person who took these photos hadn't been paying attention or didn't think those warnings were important.

The photos would have been quite a shock to the average vanilla person who was not used to seeing pictures of a fellow employee and bank executive flogging a semi-nude woman chained to a spanking bench. She printed the photos on her office printer and took them to the CEO of the bank.

Monday morning, I was called into the CEO's office and shown the photos. He said, "Mike, I love you like a son, but I'm afraid I am going to have to ask you to resign. I've prepared a generous severance package for you, which I hope you'll find agreeable." He handed me an envelope and said, "Clean out your desk. We'll escort you out."

And just like that, my career in banking was over. All because someone thought it would be *cool* to post kinky pictures of me on Facebook.

**Question #61:** If this collar symbolizes our commitment to each other, then what specifically do you think that commitment is?

**Follow-up questions:**

Does your commitment to me differ in any way from my commitment to you? Why or why not?

What would constitute a violation or failure to meet that commitment?

**Why it's important:**

Entering into a collared D/s relationship without a real understanding of what the commitment really means is a sure recipe for disaster.

**How to interpret his answer:**

This is a question that deserves far more attention than can be given to it in a single discussion. This topic should be revisited again and again, as your relationship progresses. Expectations, wants, and needs have a way of evolving over time.

**What you should do about it:**

Compare his responses with your observations of his current behavior, and with what you know about his previous relationships. Take note of his responses and preserve them for the future. There may come a time when you may want to refer back to them for clarification, or to assess whether the two of you are getting closer to your goals or further away from them.

A D/s relationship contract may be useful for this purpose, even though they are *not* legal contracts and are completely unenforceable in court. Even so, a contract *can* be useful as a reminder of what the two of you agreed to at the start of your relationship and a standard by which the health of your relationship can be evaluated in the future.

## My Two Cents:

If your relationship is in trouble, a collar won't make it better. Let me say it one more time, just to be absolutely clear about this: A collar won't fix *anything*, and neither will a slave contract.

I found myself making this point to a casual friend just a few days ago. She wanted my opinion on a slave contract that she was drafting in anticipation of being re-collared by her former Master, who had released her several months ago but now wanted her back.

She told me, "We had a contract before, but I got hurt pretty bad. I'm hoping we get it right this time. We have trust issues that need to be resolved, and there are lots of financial questions that need to be addressed in the contract, too."

I asked, "What is it you need from me, exactly?"

She replied, "Well, I want a contract that will ensure that I don't get hurt again. I want a contract that prevents him from cheating on me like he did before and spells out the limits of our financial responsibilities. Could you just help me out by taking a look at it and telling me what you think?"

I shook my head. "No contract on earth is going to be able to do that. Trust me; the problems in your past relationship had nothing to do with the wording of your slave contract. It had everything to do with your partner's real intentions. If he wanted to screw you over again, not even a legally binding contract would be able to prevent it, much less an unenforceable, illegal slave contract. If you're really that worried about him hurting you again, then why in the world are you falling for the exact same bullcrap a second time?"

She had no answer that she was willing to share with me.

**Question #62:** Where do we go from here?

**Follow-up questions:**

What's the next step or next phase of our relationship?

How do we get to where we eventually want to be, and what is your projected timeline?

Who do you expect will accompany us on that journey?

How will this make us happier?

What are the potential pitfalls or roadblocks we should be prepared for?

**Why it's important:**

If you don't know where you're going, chances are slim that you'll ever get there. You may not have a detailed road map, but it's critical that you have some idea where you'd like to be and what you'd like to be doing a year, five years, or even ten years down the road.

**How to interpret his answer:**

Ask yourself probing questions about his responses to this set of questions as you evaluate what he tells you. Is his vision for your joint future realistic or pure fantasy? Does his vision describe someplace where you want to be? Can you see a clear path leading to the accomplishment of those goals? How willing is he to compromise on any of his ideas about the future? How willing are you?

**What you should do about it:**

There's an old saying: Failing to plan is planning to fail. If your shared future is something he hasn't given any thought at all to yet, now would a good time to start.

The *good* news is, now you get to do it as a team.

**My Two Cents:**

I have always been a big fan of comedian Steve Martin. I especially liked his comedy bit entitled, "How to Be a Millionaire and Never Pay Taxes!"

According to Steve, the first step in the process was, *"Get a million dollars!"* Step two, which he instructs you to implement once the Internal Revenue Service asks why you didn't pay your taxes, is to say, "I forgot!"

Sure, it's technically a plan, but hardly a good one.

Sound like anyone you know?

# Chapter 5: Epilogue

You now have in your relationship tool kit a wide selection of soul searching topics and follow-up questions designed to help pave the way to a happier, more fulfilling D/s dynamic. You've probably come up with plenty of additional questions of your own as you've perused these pages and contemplated the topics we've touched upon. If so, good for you!

I hope you will never lose sight of the fact that the overall purpose of this interview process is to help you find the right potential Dominant for you, assist in establishing a healthy and fulfilling relationship with that person, and give you some tools for maintaining and enjoying that relationship for as long as possible. Preferably, that means "happily ever after."

Contrary to popular belief, happily ever after endings really can and do happen in the D/s and BDSM lifestyles. Don't let the things you see in social media or chat rooms skew your perceptions of what the lifestyle is really like. Once you start going to local group munches or fetish events and making new friends, you'll see that this lifestyle isn't really much different from what you're already used to.

The most common reason most people have for not getting involved with their local BDSM group is the false belief that the people they'll meet there are somehow different from the general population. They are *not*. They are exactly the same people you already know and meet regularly in your day-to-day activities. Believe it or not, you are not the *only* freak in town.

Please trust me on this. Everyone has sex. Everyone has kinks. Everyone thinks they're the only ones. They're *not*. *You're* not. So, get *over* it.

The best way for you to find the right partner in this lifestyle is to get involved and meet people. It's not so scary once you realize these people are just like you. I'm always amazed when new people come to one of our local BDSM group munches and always say the same silly thing:

"Wow! You guys all seem so.... *normal!*"

Well, duh. Perhaps that's because we *are*.

The very next thing they invariably say is, "This is fun! You guys are great! It's not at *all* what I expected. I thought you people would be scary! I should have done this years ago!"

Yes, you *should* have! And why didn't you? Is it because you're afraid someone might find out that you like sex? Is it because you've been brainwashed into thinking that it's not okay to admit to being who and what you really are? Surely, it isn't because you enjoy being *lonely*.

Put your big-girl panties on and get out there and make some new friends.

*You can do this.*

The key to success in finding the right Dominant for you will be a matter of going in with your eyes wide open, and having realistic expectations.

If you think you are going to find "Mr. Right" in your first interview, you're simply wrong. Realistically speaking, your odds are closer to one in fifty. Yes, you're going to have to kiss a lot of frogs to find your prince. Not only will that require a great deal of raw determination, intestinal fortitude, and lots of patience, but you're going to have to learn to get good at a brand new sport: the frog toss.

Just because someone is interested in you does not make him or her right for you. Get over the notion that you are unworthy and therefore anyone who shows any interest in you at all somehow deserves your attention. They do *not*.

Cast a wide net. Talk to a lot of prospects. Be perfectly willing to move on when someone does not match the profile of what you are looking for in a Dominant. Do *not* settle for someone who will ultimately be incompatible with you. You're just asking for heartbreak and hassles in the future that you could easily have avoided by doing the right thing right now.

One reason so many submissives have a difficult time finding the right Dominant is simple, really. They spend most of their time on the *wrong ones*. They get wrapped up in the drama and the intrigue and that whole business of teaching Mr. Wrong a lesson that they leave no time at all for Mr. Right to get his foot in the door.

You don't owe Mr. Wrong a damn thing. You don't owe him an explanation for why he isn't right for you. You don't owe him a response to his repeated efforts at sending you pictures of his genitalia. You don't owe him a date, or a nude picture, or a blowjob, or your mother's tuna casserole recipe. You don't owe him anything at *all*.

He is Mr. Wrong. Every minute you spend dealing with Mr. Wrong is a minute you'll never get back and a minute that Mr. Right is forced to focus *his* attention on someone *else*.

In the business world, there is something called the 80-20 rule. Most businesses spend the great majority of their time focused on the 80% of their customers who are the *most* trouble and the *least* profitable, while virtually ignoring their most loyal and profitable customers.

The squeaky wheel may get the grease, but focusing solely on squeaky wheels is an extremely poor way to do business.

The world's most successful and profitable businesses spend 80% of their time, resources, and energy on the *most* profitable 20% of their clientele. And it pays off very handsomely for them.

Are you spending all your time on the frogs, instead of the princes? The moment you realize that someone isn't right for you, you should *move on.* Don't bother trying to teach him a lesson. Don't waste time trying to get him to admit that he was wrong. Don't spend the next three days telling everyone you know that he's a *douchebag.* Don't pine over him. Don't second-guess your decision. Don't keep tabs on him. Don't doodle his name or daydream about what could have been.

Just. Move. *On.*

Look forward, not backward. He's out there, somewhere. Cast a wide net and ask the right questions until you finally find him.

Then, *keep* him.

# Appendix A: Bonus Questions

Here are some simple *"either-or"* questions that can be used to provide you and your prospective Dominant with an entertaining way to learn about each other's likes, dislikes, and preferences. To add a little depth to the discussion, you might even want to consider following up each choice with, *"Why* is that your preference?"

Asking questions or answering questions?

Coke or Pepsi?

Vanilla or chocolate?

Boxers or briefs?

McDonald's or Burger King?

Tea or coffee?

Phone call or text?

Comedy movie or horror movie?

Summer or winter?

Rock, rap, or country music?

White bread or wheat?

Coffee or tea?

Black & white or color photographs?

Drawings or paintings?

Dresses or skirts?

Books or movies?

Chinese or Italian?

Early bird or night owl?

Introvert or extrovert?

Hugs or kisses?

Hunting or fishing?

Meat or vegetables?

Spring or fall?

City or country?

PC or Mac?

Sunshine or tanning booth?

Cake or pie?

Ice cream or yogurt?

Ketchup or mustard?

Sweet pickles or dill pickles?

Heels or sandals?

Silver or gold?

Jazz or classical music?

Singing or dancing?

Male or female vocalists?

Chess or checkers?

Board games or video games?

Wine or beer?

Freckles or dimples?

Aerobic or resistance exercise?

Baseball or basketball?

Crossword puzzles or sudoku?

Newspaper or internet news?

Facial hair or clean shaven?

Crushed ice or cubed?

Skiing or snowboarding?

Bracelet or necklace?

Fruit or vegetables?

Sausage or bacon?

Scrambled or fried?

Dark chocolate or white chocolate?

Tattoos or piercings?

Antique or new furniture?

Dress up or dress down?

Cowboys or aliens?

Cats or dogs?

Pancakes or waffles?

Bond or Bourne?

Sci-Fi or fantasy?

Numbers or letters?

Star Wars or Star Trek?

Country fair or amusement park?

Fame or wealth?

Washing dishes or doing laundry?

Snakes or sharks?

Orange juice or apple juice?

Sunrise or sunset?

Slacker or over-achiever?

Pen or pencil?

Peanut butter or jelly?

Grammys or Oscars?

Detailed or abstract?

Multiple choice or essay questions?

Adventurous or cautious?

Saver or spender?

Glasses or contacts?

Laptop or desktop?

Classic or modern?

Personal chef or personal fitness trainer?

Internet or cell phone?

Curly hair or straight hair?

Blondes or brunettes?

Morning shower or evening shower?

Spicy or mild?

Marvel or DC?

Paying a mortgage or paying rent?

Sky diving or bungee jumping?

Oreos or Chips Ahoy?

Jello or pudding?

Popsicle or ice cream?

Truth or dare?

Roller coaster or Ferris wheel?

Denim or leather?

Stripes or solids?

Bagels or muffins?

Beads or pearls?

Hardwood or carpet?

Bright colors or pastels?

To be older or younger than you are now?

Raisins or nuts?

Picnic or a nice restaurant?

Long hair or short hair?

Fiction or non-fiction?

Heroes or heroines?

Smoking or non-smoking?

# Appendix B: Glossary

"When I use a word,' Humpty Dumpty said in rather a scornful tone, 'it means just what I choose it to mean — neither more nor less."

"The question is," said Alice, "whether you can make words mean so many different things."

"The question is," said Humpty Dumpty, "which is to be master. That's *all."*

### # # #

**BDSM**. Bondage, Discipline, Sadism, Masochism. Some revisionists like to posit that the DS in BDSM can also stand for Domination and Submission, but it is my belief that this confuses the public by blurring the line between BDSM and D/s.

**Bottom.** A term used in both the BDSM and gay lifestyles to refer to a person in a submissive, passive, receiving or obedient role. The term is usually applied to describe a person's actions and behaviors demonstrated at any given moment in time, rather than his or her deep-seated character and thought-processes. In a nutshell, one's actions may make him a bottom, while one's character may make him a submissive. There is often some overlap and it is entirely possible to be a submissive who is not in the role of a bottom at any given time or circumstance.

**Brat.** A submissive who is generally well-behaved, but has made misbehavior, teasing, and limited kinds of defiance or disobedience an integral part of her D/s dynamic, preferably with the full awareness and at least the implied approval of her Dominant.

**Collar.** Collars are viewed by those in the D/s lifestyle in much the same way that rings are considered by those outside of the lifestyle. Just as a ring can symbolize anything from friendship to marriage, or have no symbolism whatsoever, so too can a collar. A collar can be comprised of just about anything, to include a ribbon around the neck, an actual pet collar, custom designed fetish-wear, or even a traditional necklace that only you know the significance of. A collar is simply what the people involved agree that it is, nothing more, nothing less. When a Dominant no longer feels his submissive is worthy of the collar, the submissive may be "released," meaning the collar is revoked.

**Consent.** Consent, for BDSM purposes, refers to the informed agreement to engage in an activity, scene or relationship, assuming that all parties have a mutual understanding of what is meant by the agreement. Evidence or proof of a partner's prior consent may be difficult to prove after the fact, which can be problematic considering the fact that it is typically the critical factor when it comes to criminal charges such as assault, sodomy, and rape. Even so, documenting consent is a relatively rare thing in the BDSM lifestyle.

**Cow/Pig.** A submissive is one who enjoys being treated like a domesticated farm animal, and thrives on humiliation, degradation, and abuse from her Dominant and focuses on the real or imagined unattractiveness of the submissive.

**Discipline.** Traditionally the "D" in BDSM. Generally speaking, it refers to various forms of corporal punishment, such as spanking, caning, beating, flogging, whipping, or slapping. In a more subtle sense, discipline can also refer to the mental discipline required to be a good Dominant or submissive, which sometimes requires a disciplined mindset that allows a person to resist his or her natural impulses.

**Domestic**. Often referred to as a service submissive. Domestics are expected to perform household duties such as cooking, cleaning, childcare, chauffeuring, and yard work. He or she is typically expected to be sexually available to the Dom, his other submissives, or guests.

**Dominant**. One who acts in a domineering or authoritative role in life, and especially in relationships. A Dominant may be a "true Dominant" in the sense that this trait is firmly hard-wired into his psyche and he simply doesn't know any other way to be, or he may be acting out a role, whether consciously or unconsciously. A Dominant is defined primarily by his need to control his environment and personal interactions and his skill at being able to do so.

**Domme**. A female Dominant, sometimes referred to as a Dominatrix or Mistress. Generally speaking, a Domme may refer to any female Dominant, however, outside of the D/s lifestyle, the stereotype typically fits the FemDom Mistress. The correct pronunciation of *Domme* is identical to *Dom*.

**D/s**. Domination and submission, a phrase which describes a *relationship dynamic* that exists between two or more individuals in a loving relationship. While D/s refers to the dynamic, it defines *who you are in relation to the individual who is your partner*. Who you are at work, or with your children, or around casual friends is *irrelevant* to this paradigm.

**Ineffable**. A somewhat archaic word, meaning "incapable of being adequately described." It was once a very trendy thing to refer to *God* as being *ineffable*. Now, often used to refer to Doms or subs who are difficult to categorize or describe.

**Kajira**. A female Gorean slave in the tradition of John Norman's series of pulp science fiction novels about the planet Gor.

**Kneeling.** Kneeling is sometimes used as a euphemism for submitting to a Dominant but is, more often than not, a reference to assuming a submissive posture by sitting on the floor on your knees. Various fetish culture sub-groups may place more or less emphasis on the significance of kneeling. Goreans, for example, teach slaves to assume a series of positions on command from their Masters, many of which are kneeling positions.

**Lesser God Dominant.** A Dominant who thrives on the worship of his submissives. This worship, which can sometimes take the form of highly ritualistic activities and behaviors, exists for the ego gratification of the Lesser God and the practice their own home-grown religion.

**Little**. A Little is a submissive who finds joy in embracing her inner child. This dynamic often involves behaving, speaking, dressing in a child-like manner, or engaging in typical child-appropriate activities, and may or may not involve sex or other adult-appropriate themes. Also referred to often as *babygirls or lolitas*.

**Master.** Master is an appellation, title, or even a term of endearment which may be used by a slave or submissive for his or her Dominant. Some Dominants consider Master to be a generic synonym for Dominant, although that practice is generally most prevalent in the Gorean subculture. Other Dominants reserve the use of the title of Master only to those whom they have collared.

**Misandry / Misandrist**. Hatred or dislike of men as a class; not necessarily targeting men as individuals.

**Munch Group.** A local kink-related group that meets regularly for coffee or a meal in a vanilla setting (usually a restaurant) purely for social purposes. A munch group may also have BDSM events or play parties, but those are *not* the same as *munches* and, generally speaking, strangers are not allowed to attend them unless they've been vetted or vouched for by a trusted member.

**Novice**. Someone who has very recently discovered and become excited about the D/s or BDSM lifestyle and has decided that he or she badly wants to be a part of it *at any cost.*

**Painslut**. An extreme masochist who enjoys or is aroused by sensations of intense and/or prolonged pain.

**Pet**. A Pet submissive assumes the role of a cherished animal companion to her Dominant, who typically assumes the role of an owner, caretaker, trainer, breeder, or rider. The pet roles *generally* fall into three categories: kittens, puppies, and ponies.

**Polyamory.** The practice or ability to love more than one person at a time; from the Latin poly (many) and amor (love). Just because polyamory is relatively common in the D/s lifestyle doesn't mean that people in the lifestyle are any better at it than anyone else. It is a profoundly difficult thing to be successfully polyamorous in any relationship, D/s or otherwise.

**Polyandry.** Refers to a polyamorous relationship in which a woman has more than one male partner. It is typically used to describe a polygamous or plural marriage consisting of a wife with two or more husbands.

**Polyfidelous.** The practice of being faithful to more than one partner, usually in a polyamorous relationship, is called polyfidelity. For example, a polyamorous Dominant with two submissives may choose to be polyfidelous to his two partners, not engaging in intimate relations with anyone else. This may or may not include BDSM fetish-play, as many people in the BDSM lifestyle do not consider such activity as "intimate." Ultimately, the meaning of polyfidelity must be mutually agreed upon by the individuals in that relationship.

**Polygyny.** Refers to a polyamorous relationship in which a man has more than one female partner. It is typically used to describe a polygamous or plural marriage consisting of a husband with two or more wives.

**Primal.** A person who embraces his or her animalistic or primal instincts. Primals are often neither inherently dominant nor submissive by nature. Primals tend to prefer nontraditional poly relationships patterned on the pack or pride dynamic, similar to that of wolves and lions. Primals do treat dominance and submission as a significant part of their interactions with others, but it is something that is fluid and spontaneous, and often established in an ad-hoc, spur of the moment fashion upon meeting someone for the first time.

**Pseudo-sub.** Someone who may be fairly new to the lifestyle and truly believes that he or she is a submissive, despite overwhelming evidence to the contrary.

**Slave.** A submissive who cultivates and enjoys the illusion that he or she has no free will. The fact that this is an illusion should surprise no one, since the foundation of any D/s relationship is always consent. Many in the lifestyle consider this a form of consensual non-consent.

**Submissive.** A person who finds joy and fulfillment in service or submission to another. She is defined by the relationship dynamic that exists between the submissive and her Dominant, *not* by any *other* characteristics or behaviors that she might display elsewhere in her day-to-day life.

**Switch.** The *classic switch* is someone who is *submissive* to one person (or category of persons) while, at the same time, dominant towards another. A good example is the alpha submissive in a poly

Dominant's household, who takes responsibility for the training and supervision of the other submissives in the same house. The contemporary meaning of switch has evolved to refer to a person who can change his or her D/s or BDSM orientation at will.

**Top.** A Top is someone who situationally or temporarily assumes the dominant, leading, or aggressive role as part of an activity which is usually, but not necessarily limited to, a BDSM scene. A Top may or may not be a Dominant. Conversely and less commonly, a Dominant is not always a Top.

**Topping from the Bottom.** A submissive's practice of manipulating or influencing the decisions or behavior of a Dominant. This behavior by the submissive can be overt, purposeful, and conscious, or it can be covert, subtle, and unconscious. It is sometimes accomplished with the full knowledge and approval of the Dominant. Other times, the Dominant may be oblivious to it, even if everyone else can see it. The brat sub is the type of submissive that is most commonly associated with this sort of behavior, but in reality, it is practiced by all kinds of submissives, in every category of D/s relationship.

**Total Power Exchange (TPE).** Total Power Exchange refers to the notion that a D/s relationship or BDSM scene involves not just a surrender of power from one individual to another, but an *exchange* of power. This exchange may involve different kinds of power, and is likely to be asymmetrical, but is an *exchange* nevertheless.

**Vanilla.** Term used by those in the D/s, BDSM or fetish lifestyles to describe those outside of the lifestyle. It is generally used in the sense that anything that is vanilla flavored (i.e. ice cream) is considered to be unexciting or bland. The term vanilla is rarely used as a serious pejorative or insult, though some people will occasionally choose to interpret it as such.

# Appendix C: About the Author

Michael Makai is the best-selling author of Domination & Submission: The BDSM Relationship Handbook, The Warrior Princess Submissive, 62Q: Sixty-two Questions For Your Dominant, and The BDSM Coloring Book.

Michael has been a lifestyle Dominant for 37 years, a behind-the-scenes mentor and educator on BDSM and D/s for decades, and has been active in dozens of fetish lifestyle organizations in Europe and the United States. Michael believes that one of the keys to understanding the lifestyle and the people in it is to be able to recognize the very distinct differences between BDSM, which is something you do, and D/s, which is a relationship dynamic.

Michael is a combat veteran and a retired senior Army noncommissioned officer with over 20 years of active military service. He has worked as a marketing consultant, banker, freelance writer, magazine publisher, internet service provider, and a stock market trader. He is an incorrigible word-maker-upperer who enjoys skiing, traveling, playing Scrabble, and raising koi.

He currently resides near Wichita Falls, Texas.

Made in the USA
San Bernardino, CA
28 February 2017